P9-EEM-193

POCKET GUIDE TO

Gerontologic Assessment

Annette Giesler Lueckenotte, MS, RN, CS

Gerontologic Nurse Practitioner
Alexian Brothers Senior Health Center
St. Louis, Missouri

Third Edition

Illustrated

Mosby

St. Louis Baltimore Boston Carlsbad
Chicago Minneapolis New York Philadelphia Portland
London Milan Sydney Tokyo Toronto

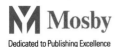

Mosby
Dedicated to Publishing Excellence

A Times Mirror Company

Publisher: Nancy L. Coon
Editor: Michael S. Ledbetter
Developmental Editor: Laurie K. Muench
Editorial Assistant: Dina Shourd
Project Manager: John Rogers
Production Editor: Jeanne Genz
Designer: Yael Kats
Manufacturing Manager: Linda Ierardi

Third Editon

Printed in the United States of America
Composition by The Clarinda Company
Printing/binding by R.R. Donnelley & Sons Company

Mosby, Inc.
11830 Westline Industrial Drive
St. Louis, Missouri 63146

Library of Congress Cataloging in Publication Data

Lueckenotte, Annette Giesler.
    Pocket guide to gerontologic assessment / Annette Giesler
Lueckenotte. —3rd ed.
        p. cm.
    Includes index.
    ISBN 0-8151-2799-5
    1. Geriatric nursing—Handbooks, manuals, ect.   2. Nursing
assessment—handbooks, manuals, etc. I. Title.
    [DNLM: 1. Nursing Assessment—handbooks.   2. Physical Examination-
-in old age—handbooks.   3. Geriatric Nursing—methods—handbooks.
WY 49 L948p 1997]
RC954.L83   1997
610.73′65—dc21
DNLM/DLC
for Library of Congress   97-34218
                                                                    CIP

97 98 99 00 01 / 9 8 7 6 5 4 3 2 1

Reviewers

Karen Lamb, ND, RN, CS
Assistant Professor/Practitioner Teacher
Rush University College of Nursing
Chicago, Illinois

Susan Sanders, MSN, CRNP
Adult and Geriatric Nurse Practitioner
Memorial Community Clinic
Midland, Texas

Lynn Sivertsen, MSN, RN, CS
Assistant Professor/Practitioner Teacher
Rush University College of Nursing
Chicago, Illinois

Preface

The third edition of *Pocket Guide to Gerontologic Nursing* has been designed and written to serve as a practical guide for nurses assessing the health status of older adults in a variety of traditional and nontraditional settings. This book is intended to guide the nurse in the performance of a basic, comprehensive health assessment that covers all body systems. The organization of the guide provides a quick, ready reference when conducting focused assessment related to a specific body system, or when conducting a complete health assessment. Additional content in this third edition includes a chapter on nutritional assessment; a section in Chapter 2 identifying drugs that may influence assessment of the older client; sample documentation boxes at the end of each of the body system chapters that show how to record the collected subjective and objective data in an organized format; and a section in Chapter 16 on foot assessment.

The first two chapters continue to emphasize the nursing focus of health assessment, while they also address the special considerations affecting older adult assessment. Suggestions are included for tailoring the nursing assessment based on the unique differences of this age group. The sample health history format in Chapter 2 can be adapted for use with clients at any point on the health-illness continuum. Samples of selected standardized tools to augment traditional clinical assessment are also provided. The focus of Chapter 3 is on fundamental physical assessment skills, and there are also guidelines to consider when conducting an examination of the older adult. Chapter 4 is a new addition, featuring the components of nutritional assessment specific to the older adult.

Chapters 5 through 17 concern the assessment of the body systems. Each of these chapters begins with a brief illustrated overview of relevant anatomy and physiology. The method of physical examination is presented in an orderly, easy-to-follow two-column format. The first column identifies the examination sequence and describes pertinent techniques and instrumentation. The second column identifies normal age-related findings and variations of normal findings and highlights deviations from normal. Photographs and illustrations of older persons enhance the written descriptions; figures and tables serve to synthesize information for easier access. Some of these chapters close with an example of a health-promoting client-teaching topic relevant to that body system. This edition includes a sample write-up of a complete history and physical examination as an appendix. Other appendices include the latest AHCPR guidelines on urinary incontinence and pressure ulcers, as well as some guidelines for older adult laboratory values.

The purpose of older adult assessment is to determine the older person's response to actual or potential health problems in view of the identified strengths and limitations, so that effective and appropriate nursing interventions can be delivered to promote optimal functioning and prevent disability and dependence. Careful consideration of the interrelationships between physical and psychosocial health conditions is of critical importance when caring for older persons. Nurses caring for this population must use a sound aged-specific approach to assessment as the foundation for therapeutic nursing care. It is my hope that this book will expand your knowledge and enable you to meet the challenge of providing aged-appropriate care.

I would like to acknowledge the support and assistance of my editor, Michael Ledbetter, and my developmental editor, Laurie Muench, in producing this revision.

Annette Giesler Lueckenotte

Contents

1 Nursing Assessment of the Older Person, 1

2 The Interview: Obtaining the Health History, 15

3 Physical Assessment, 54

4 Nutritional Assessment, 62

5 General Survey and Mental Status Assessment, 88

6 Assessment of Integument, 95

7 Assessment of the Head, Face, and Neck, 118

8 Assessment of the Eyes, 131

9 Assessment of the Ears, Nose, and Throat, 150

10 Assessment of the Breasts, 179

11 Assessment of the Thorax and Lungs, 194

12 Assessment of the Heart and Vascular System, 214

13 Assessment of the Abdomen, 244

14   Assessment of Male Genitalia, 266

15   Assessment of Female Genitalia, 277

16   Assessment of the Musculoskeletal System, 304

17   Assessment of the Neurologic System, 326

APPENDIXES
A   Sample Health History and Physical Examination Write-Up, 349

B   Older Adult Laboratory Values, 358

C   Managing Acute and Chronic Urinary Incontinence, 360

D   Pressure Ulcers in Adults: Prediction and Prevention, 390

Nursing Assessment of the Older Person

1

Nursing Foundations

The nursing process is a problem-solving process that provides the organizational framework for the provision of nursing care. Assessment, the crucial foundation on which the remaining steps of the process are built, includes the collection and analysis of data and results in a nursing diagnosis. A nursing-focused assessment is crucial to the determination of nursing diagnoses that are amenable to nursing intervention. Unless the approach to assessment maintains a nursing focus, the subsequent planning, implementation, and evaluation steps of the nursing process cannot be carried out.

A nursing focus evolves from an awareness and understanding of the purpose of nursing. This purpose, as defined in the American Nurses Association's publication *Nursing: A Social Policy Statement,* "is the diagnosis and treatment of human responses to actual or potential health problems" (American Nurses Association, 1980). This definition directs the nurse to gather data that will assist in determining the client's response to actual or potential health problems. A comprehensive, nursing-focused assessment of responses reflects the client's ability to meet physical and psychosocial needs. Client responses that reveal an inability to meet these needs indicate a need for nursing care.

Nursing-focused assessment of older people occurs in the traditional settings of the home, hospital, or long-term care institution, as well as in nontraditional settings such as senior centers, apartment buildings, or nursing group practices. The setting dictates the way data collection and analysis should be managed to serve clients best. Although the approach to nursing-focused assessment of older adult clients may vary with regard to the setting, the purpose remains that of determining the older person's response to actual or potential health problems. Specifically, the purpose of older adult assessment is to identify client strengths and limitations so that effective and appropriate interventions can be delivered to promote optimal functioning and to prevent disability and dependence.

Gerontologic nurses recognize that assessing older adult clients involves complex and varied issues. Careful, nursing-focused assessment based on a sound, gerontologic knowledge base is essential for recognition of client responses that reflect unmet needs. Many frameworks and tools are available to guide the nurse in assessing the older adult. Regardless of the framework or tool used, the nurse should collect the data while observing the following key principles: (1) using an individual, person-centered approach; (2) viewing the client as a participant in health monitoring and treatment; and (3) emphasizing the client's functional ability.

Special Considerations Affecting Assessment

Nursing assessment of an older adult client is a complex and challenging process that must take into account the following points to ensure an age-specific approach.

Interrelationship Between Physical and Psychosocial Aspects of Aging

The health of people of all ages is subject to the influence of any number and kind of physical and psychosocial variables within the environment. The balance that is achieved within that environment of many variables influences a person's health status. For the older person, factors such as reduced ability to respond to stress, increased frequency and multiplicity of loss, and the general changes associated with normal aging can combine to place the aged client at high risk for loss of functional ability. Consider the following case, which illustrates how the interaction of selected physical and psychosocial variables can seriously compromise function.

Mrs. S., 78, arrived in the emergency room after sustaining a hip fracture resulting from a fall in her home. She had been found lying on the floor of her bathroom 7 hours after the fall, confused and incontinent of urine. Because of the emergent nature of the admission, Mrs. S. did not have any personal belongings with her, including her hearing aid and glasses. Buck's traction was applied to the affected extremity on admission to the nursing division. Twelve hours later she had surgery to repair the fracture, and then returned to a different nursing division.

Two days postoperatively, pain control remained a problem despite the nurses' attempts to administer narcotic analgesics regularly. An antipsychotic was also administered for persistent confusion. Mrs. S. became increasingly anorexic and unwilling to participate in physical therapy. She slept long hours during the day and was found crying frequently when awake.

Table 1-1 depicts the many serious consequences of the interacting variables in this case. A word of caution: undue emphasis should not be placed on individual decrements. In fact, it is imperative that the gerontologic nurse search for the client's

Table 1-1   Effect of selected variables on functional status

Variable	Effect
Visual and auditory loss	Apathy
	Confusion, disorientation
	Dependency, loss of control
Multiple strange and unfamiliar environments	Confusion
	Dependency, loss of control
	Sleep disturbance
	Relocation stress
Acute musculoskeletal injury	Mobility impairment
	Dependency, loss of control
	Sleep disturbance
Altered pharmacokinetics and pharmacodynamics	Persistent confusion
	Drug toxicity
	Potential for further mobility impairment, loss of function, and altered patterns of bowel and bladder elimination
	Loss of appetite, in turn affecting wound healing, bowel function, and energy level; dehydration
	Sleep disturbance (oversedation)

strengths and abilities and build the plan of care on these. However, in a situation such as this, the nurse should be aware of the potential for the consequences illustrated here. A single problem is not likely, since multiple conditions are often superimposed on one another. In addition, the cause of one problem may best be understood in view of the accompanying problems. Careful consideration, then, of the interrelationships between the physical and psychosocial aspects of a particular client situation is essential.

Nature of Disease and Disability, and Effects on Functional Status

Aging does not necessarily result in disease and disability. Although the prevalence of chronic disease increases with age, most older people remain functionally independent. Assessment of physical and psychosocial function can provide valuable clues to the effect of a disease on functional status. Also, the self-report of vague signs and symptoms such as lethargy, incontinence, decreased appetite, and weight loss can be indicators of functional impairment.

Declining organ and system function and diminishing physiologic reserve with advancing age are well documented in the literature. Such normal changes of aging may make the body more susceptible to disease and disability. It can be difficult for the nurse to differentiate normal age-related findings from indicators of disease or disability. In fact, it is not uncommon for nurses and older adults alike to mistakenly attribute vague signs and symptoms to normal aging changes or just "growing old." However, it is imperative that the nurse make the determination of what is "normal" versus what may be an indicator of disease or disability so that treatable conditions are not disregarded.

Ignoring the older adult's vague symptomatology exposes the client to an increased risk of physical frailty. Physical frailty, the impairments in physical abilities needed to live independently, is a major contributor to the need for long-term care. Therefore it is essential to investigate nonspecific signs and symptoms to determine whether there are any possible underlying conditions that contribute to frailty (National Institute on Aging, 1991).

Decreased Efficiency of Homeostatic Mechanisms

Declining physiologic function and increased prevalence of disease, particularly in the oldest old (age 85 years and older), are in part a result of a reduction in the body's ability to respond to stress through all of its homeostatic mechanisms, most importantly the immune system. The older person's adaptive reserves are reduced and their homeostatic mechanisms weakened; these factors result in a decreased ability to respond to illness and disease.

The immune system, as the body's major defense against illness and disease, reveals a decreased ability to provide protection with aging. Although scientists have attempted to identify which age-related immune system changes cause the decline in immunocompetence, it has been difficult to do so, since immunocompetence is affected by multiple other factors (Bramlett, 1996).

Increasing consideration also has been given in recent years to the potential impact of psychosocial stress on the older adult's immune system. This growing consideration, coupled with the knowledge about factors affecting physiologic immunocompetence, has potential clinical relevance that is a current source of investigation and controversy (Hillhouse and Adler, 1991). The reader is referred to an immunology text for a more complete discussion of the effect of aging on the immune response.

The important point is that older adults often encounter profound and repeated losses; the time between the occurrences of these losses is often short, resulting in an inadequate time period for resolution and return to a baseline state. Older adult clients have less ability than younger people to cope with assaults such as infection, blood loss, a high-tech environment, or loss of a significant person. The gerontologic nurse therefore has an obligation to assess older adults for the presence of both physical and psychosocial stressors and for their physical and emotional manifestations.

Lack of Standards for Health and Illness Norms

Determining an older adult's physical and psychosocial health status is not easy because norms for health and illness are always being redefined. Established standards for what is normal versus abnormal are changing as more scientific studies are conducted and the knowledge base is expanded.

One area where recent study is changing how health care providers interpret normal versus abnormal is with laboratory values. Relying on established norms for laboratory values when analyzing an older adult's assessment data could lead to incorrect conclusions. A fasting blood glucose of 70 mg/100 ml may be within the normal range for a young adult, but an older person with that same level may experience significant symptoms of hypoglycemia (see Appendix B). Polypharmacy and the multiplicity of illness and disease are only two variables that may affect laboratory data interpretation in the older adult.

In addition, there are no definitive aging norms for many pathologic conditions. For example, controversy has existed over what constitutes isolated systolic hypertension (ISH) in older people. Is a high systolic pressure simply a function of age and therefore harmless, or does it require treatment? Recent studies (Frolich, 1990) have shown that cardiovascular morbidity and mortality in older people have been reduced with therapy. As more studies are conducted in this area and others, norms will continue to be redefined.

Landmarks for human growth and development are well established for infancy through "middlescence," whereas few norms are defined for older adulthood. Developmental norms that have been described for later life categorize all older persons in the "over 65" age group. However, one could argue from a developmental perspective that as great a difference exists among persons aged 65, 75, 85, and 95 years as it does among children aged 2, 3, 4, and 5 years. In fact, given the demographic facts and predictions, there exists a very pressing need to know the developmental characteristics of older people for each decade of life.

To compensate for the lack of definitive standards, the nurse should first assume heterogeneity rather than homogeneity when caring for older people. It is crucial to respect the uniqueness of each person's life experiences and to preserve the individuality created by those experiences. The older person's experiences represent a rich and vast background that the nurse can use to develop an individualized plan of care. Second, the nurse can compare the older person's own previous patterns of physical and psychosocial health and function with the current status, using the individual as the standard (Matteson and McConnell, 1988). Finally, the nurse must have a complete and current knowledge base and skills in gerontologic nursing to apply to each individual older adult client situation.

Altered Presentation of and Response to Specific Diseases

With advanced age, the body does not respond as vigorously to injury or disease because of diminished physiologic reserve. It is important to note that the diminished reserve poses no particular problems for most older people as they carry out their daily routines. However, in times of physical and emotional stress, it causes older people to not always exhibit the expected, or "classic," signs and symptoms. The characteristic presentation of illness in older adults is more commonly one of blunted or atypical signs and symptoms.

The atypical presentation of illness can be displayed in various ways. For example, the signs and symptoms may be modified in some way, as in the case of pneumonia, when an older adult may exhibit a dry cough instead of the classic productive cough. Also, the presenting signs and symptoms may be totally unrelated to the actual problem, such as the confusion that may accompany a urinary tract infection. Finally, the expected signs and symptoms may not be present at all, as in the case of a myocardial infarction that includes no chest pain. All of these atypical presentations challenge the nurse to conduct careful and thorough assessments and analyses of symptoms to ensure appropriate treatment. Again, a simple and safe strategy is to compare the presenting signs and symptoms with the older adult's normal baseline (Table 1-2).

Cognitive impairment

As can be seen from Table 1-2, pp. 8-9, delirium is one of the most common manifestations of illness in the older adult, representing a wide variety of potential problems. Delirium, confusion, mental status changes, and cognitive changes are some of the terms used to describe one of the most common manifestations of illness in old age. Foreman (1986) advocates use of the term *acute confusional state* (ACS) to describe ". . . an organic brain syndrome characterized by transient, global cognitive impairment of abrupt onset and relatively brief duration, accompanied by diurnal fluctuation of simultaneous disturbances of the sleep-wake cycle, psychomotor behavior, attention and affect." Unfortunately, the ageist views of many health care providers cause them to believe that an ACS is a normal, expected outcome of aging, thus robbing the older adult of a complete and thorough workup of this syndrome. The nurse as the advocate for the older person may need to remind other team members that a sudden change in cognitive function is often the result of illness, *not* aging. Knowing the older adult's baseline mental status is key to avoid overlooking a serious illness manifesting itself as an ACS. The box on pp. 10-12 outlines the multivariate etiologies associated with an ACS that the nurse must consider during assessment. *Text continued on p. 12*

Table 1-2 How illness changes with age

Problem	Classic Presentation in Young Patient	Presentation in Elderly
Urinary tract infection	Dysuria, frequency, urgency, nocturia	Dysuria often *absent*; frequency, urgency, nocturia *sometimes* present. Incontinence, delirium, falls, and anorexia are other signs.
Myocardial infarction	Severe substernal chest pain, diaphoresis, nausea, dyspnea	Sometimes *no* chest pain, or atypical pain location such as in jaw, neck, shoulder, epigastric area. Dyspnea may or may not be present. Other signs are tachypnea, arrhythmia, hypotension, restlessness, syncope, fatigue/weakness. A fall may be a prodrome.
Bacterial pneumonia	Cough productive of purulent sputum, chills and fever, pleuritic chest pain, elevated white blood cell (WBC) count	Cough may be productive, dry, or absent; chills and fever and/or elevated WBCs also may be absent. Tachypnea, slight cyanosis, delirium, anorexia, nausea and vomiting, tachycardia may be present.
Congestive heart failure	Increased dyspnea (orthopnea, paroxysmal nocturnal dyspnea), fatigue, weight gain, pedal edema, nocturia, bibasilar crackles	All of the manifestations of young adult *and/or* anorexia, restlessness, delirium, cyanosis, falls.

Hyperthyroidism	Heat intolerance, fast pace, exophthalmos, increased pulse, hyperreflexia, tremor	Slowing down (apathetic hyperthyroidism), lethargy, weakness, depression, atrial fibrillation, and congestive heart failure.
Hypothyroidism	Weakness, fatigue, cold intolerance, lethargy, skin dryness and scaling, constipation	Often presents without overt symptoms; majority of cases are subclinical. Delirium, dementia, depression/lethargy, constipation, weight loss, and muscle weakness/unsteady gait are common.
Depression	Dysphoric mood and thoughts, withdrawal, crying, weight loss, constipation, insomnia	Any of classic symptoms *may/may not* be present. Memory and concentration problems, cognitive and behavioral changes, increased dependency, anxiety, and increased sleep. Muscle aches, abdominal pain or tightness, flatulence, nausea and vomiting, dry mouth, and headaches. Be alert for congestive heart failure, diabetes, cancer, infectious diseases, and anemia. Cardiovascular agents, anxiolytics, amphetamines, narcotics, and hormones can also play a role.

Modified from Henderson ML: Altered presentations, *Am J Nurs* 15:1104-1106, 1986.

Physiologic, Psychologic, and Environmental Etiologies of Acute Confusional States in the Hospitalized Elderly

Physiologic

A. Primary cerebral disease
   1. Nonstructural factors
      a. Vascular insufficiency—transient ischemic attacks, cerebral vascular accidents, thrombosis
      b. Central nervous system infection—acute and chronic meningitis, neurosyphilis, brain abscess
   2. Structural factors
      a. Trauma—subdural hematoma, concussion, contusion, intracranial hemorrhage
      b. Tumors—primary and metastatic
      c. Normal pressure hydrocephalus
B. Extracranial disease
   1. Cardiovascular abnormalities
      a. Decreased cardiac output states—myocardial infarction, arrhythmias, congestive heart failure, cardiogenic shock
      b. Alterations in peripheral vascular resistance—increased and decreased states
      c. Vascular occlusion—disseminated intravascular coagulopathy, emboli
   2. Pulmonary abnormalities
      a. Inadequate gas exchange states—pulmonary disease, alveolar hypoventilation
      b. Infection—pneumonias
   3. Systemic infective processes—acute and chronic
      a. Viral
      b. Bacterial—endocarditis, pyelonephritis, cystitis, mycotic
   4. Metabolic disturbances
      a. Electrolyte abnormalities—hypercalcemia, hypo- and hypernatremia, hypo- and hyperkalemia, hypo- and hyperchloremia, hyperphosphatemia
      b. Acidosis/alkalosis
      c. Hypo- and hyperglycemia
      d. Acute and chronic renal failure

B. Extracranial disease—cont'd
    4. Metabolic disturbances—cont'd
        e. Volume depletion—hemorrhage, inadequate fluid intake, diuretics
        f. Hepatic failure
        g. Porphyria
    5. Drug intoxications—therapeutic and substance abuse
        a. Misuse of prescribed medications
        b. Side effects of therapeutic medications
        c. Drug-drug interactions
        d. Improper use of over-the-counter medications
        e. Ingestion of heavy metals and industrial poisons
    6. Endocrine disturbance
        a. Hypo- and hyperthyroidism
        b. Diabetes mellitus
        c. Hypopituitarism
        d. Hypo- and hyperparathyroidism
    7. Nutritional deficiencies
        a. B vitamins
        b. Vitamin C
        c. Protein
    8. Physiologic stress—pain, surgery
    9. Alterations in temperature regulation—hypo- and hyperthermia
    10. Unknown physiologic abnormality—sometimes defined as pseudodelirium

Psychologic
    1. Severe emotional stress—postoperative states, relocation, hospitalization
    2. Depression
    3. Anxiety
    4. Pain—acute and chronic
    5. Fatigue
    6. Grief
    7. Sensory/perceptual deficits—noise, alteration in functioning of senses
    8. Mania
    9. Paranoia
    10. Situational disturbances

Continued

Physiologic, Psychologic, and Environmental
Etiologies of Acute Confusional States
in the Hospitalized Elderly—cont'd

Environmental

1. Unfamiliar environment creating a lack of meaning in the environment
2. Sensory deprivation/environmental monotony creating a lack of meaning in the environment
3. Sensory overload
4. Immobilization—therapeutic, physical, pharmacologic
5. Sleep deprivation
6. Lack of temporospatial reference points

Modified from Foreman MD: Acute confusional states in hospitalized
elderly: a research dilemma, *Nurs Res* 35:34-37, 1986.

Families and friends can be valuable sources of data regarding the onset, cause, duration, and associated symptoms of an illness that presents as an ACS. Mental status examination and functional status assessment, important components of assessment of a confused older adult client, are discussed in more detail in Chapter 2.

Tailoring the Nursing Assessment to the Older Person

The health assessment may be collected in a variety of physical settings, including hospital, home, office, clinic, day care center, and long-term care facility. Any of these settings can be adapted to be conducive to the free exchange of information between the nurse and the aged client. The overall atmosphere established by the nurse should be one that conveys trust, caring, and confidentiality.

Environmental modification made during the assessment should take into account sensory and musculoskeletal changes. The following points should be considered in preparation of the environment:

Adequate space, particularly if the client uses a mobility aid.

Minimum noise and distraction, such as that generated from television, radio, intercom, or other nearby activity.

Comfortable, sufficiently warm temperature with no drafts.

Diffuse lighting with increased illumination; avoid directional or localized light.

No glossy or highly polished surfaces, including floors, walls, ceilings, or furnishings.

Comfortable seating position that facilitates information exchange.

Proximity to a bathroom.

Available water or other preferred fluids.

Place to hang or store garments and belongings.

Absolute privacy.

Plan the assessment, taking into account the older adult's energy level, pace, and adaptability. More than one session may be necessary to complete the assessment.

Be patient, relaxed, and unhurried.

Allow the client plenty of time to respond to questions and directions.

Maximize the use of silence to allow the client time to collect thoughts before responding.

Be alert to signs of increasing fatigue, such as sighing, grimacing, irritability, leaning against objects for support, drooping of head and shoulders, and progressive slowing.

Conduct assessment during client's peak energy time, usually early in the day.

Regardless of the degree of decrement and decline an aged client may exhibit, there are assets and capabilities that allow the client to function within the limitations imposed by that decline. During the assessment, the nurse must provide an environment that gives the older adult the opportunity to demonstrate those abilities. Failure to do so could result in incorrect conclusions about the client's functional ability, which may lead to inappropriate care and treatment.

Assess more than once and at different times of day.

Measure performance under the most favorable conditions.

Take advantage of natural opportunities that would elicit assets and capabilities; collect data at times such as during bathing, grooming, and mealtime.

Ensure that assistive sensory devices (glasses, hearing aid) and mobility devices (walker, cane, prosthesis) are in place and functioning correctly.

Interview family, friends, and significant others who are involved in the client's care to validate assessment data.

Use body language, touch, eye contact, and speech to promote the client's maximum degree of participation.

Be aware of the client's emotional state and concerns; fear, anxiety, and boredom can lead to inaccurate assessment conclusions regarding functional ability.

References

American Nurses Association: *Nursing: a social policy statement,* Kansas City, Mo, 1980, American Nurses Association.

Bramlett MH: Infection. In Lueckenotte AG, editor: *Gerontologic nursing,* St Louis, 1996, Mosby.

Foreman MD: Acute confusional states in hospitalized elderly: a research dilemma, *Nurs Res* 35:34-37, 1986.

Frohlich ED: Hypertension. In Abrams WB, Berkow R, Fletcher A, editors: *Merck manual of geriatrics,* Rahway, NJ, 1990, Merck, Sharp & Dohme Research Laboratories.

Henderson ML: Altered presentations, *Am J Nurs* 15:1104-1106, 1986.

Hillhouse J, Adler C: Stress, health and immunity: a review of the literature and implications for the nursing profession, *Holistic Nurse Pract* 5(4):22-31, 1991.

Matteson MA, McConnell EJ: *Gerontological nursing: concepts and practice,* Philadelphia, 1988, WB Saunders.

Physical frailty: a reducible barrier to independence for older Americans, NIH Pub. 91-397, Bethesda, Md, 1991, National Institute on Aging.

The Interview: Obtaining the Health History

2

Adapting Interviewing Techniques

The health history and interview, as the first phase of a comprehensive health assessment, provides a subjective account of the older adult's current and past health status. The interview forms the basis of a therapeutic nurse-client relationship, in which the client's well-being is the mutual concern. The establishment of this relationship with the older client is essential to gathering useful, significant data. The data obtained from the health history alert the nurse to focus on key areas of the physical examination requiring further investigation. By talking with the nurse about health concerns, the older client's awareness of health is increased, and topics for health teaching can be identified. Finally, the process of recounting one's history in a purposeful, systematic way can have the therapeutic effect of serving as a life review.

The Interviewer

The ability of the interviewer to elicit meaningful data from the client depends on the interviewer's attitudes and stereotypes about aging and older people. The nurse must be aware of these factors because they affect nurse-client communication during the assessment.

Attitude as a feeling, value, or belief about something determines behavior. If the nurse has an attitude that characterizes older people as less healthy and alert and more dependent, then the interview structure will reflect this attitude. For example, if the nurse believes that dependence in self-care normally accompanies advanced age, the client will not be questioned about strengths and abilities. The resulting inaccurate functional assessment will do little to promote client independence.

Myths and stereotypes about older adults also can affect the nurse's questioning. For example, believing that older people do not participate in sexual relationships can result in the nurse's failure to interview the client about sexual health matters. The nurse's own anxiety and fear of personal aging, as well as a lack of knowledge regarding older people, contribute to commonly held negative attitudes, myths, and stereotypes about the aged. Gerontologic nurses have a responsibility to themselves and to their older adult clients to improve their understanding of the aging process and aging people.

To ensure a successful interview, the nurse should explain to the client the reason for the interview and give a brief overview of the format to be followed. This alleviates anxiety and uncertainty, and the client can then focus on telling the story. Another strategy that can be used in some settings is to give the client selected portions of the interview form to complete *before* meeting with the nurse. This allows clients sufficient time to recall their long life histories, thus enabling the collection of important health-related data.

Because of their long lives, older people have lengthy and often complicated histories. A goal-directed interviewing process helps the client share the pertinent information, but the tendency to reminisce may make it difficult for the client to stay focused on the topic. Guided reminiscence, however, can elicit valuable data and promote a supportive therapeutic relationship. Using such a technique helps the nurse balance the need to collect the required information with the client's need to relate what is personally important. For example, the client may relate a story about a social outing that seems irrelevant, but it may elicit important information about available resources and support systems. The interplay of the previously noted factors may necessitate more than one encounter with the client to complete the database. Setting a time limit in advance helps the client focus on the interview and aids with the problem of decreased time perception. Keeping a clock that is easy to read within view of the client may be helpful.

Because of the need to structure the interview, there is a tendency for the nurse to exhibit controlling behavior with the client.

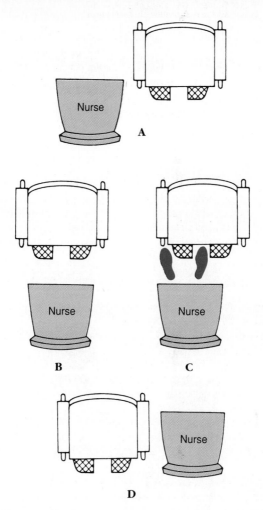

Fig. 2-1
Positions with wheelchair-bound client. **A,** One common placement of the interviewer when the client is in a wheelchair. **B,** A position for the interviewer who wants to ensure that eye contact is maintained. **C,** The best position to use with older persons in wheelchairs who are blind, hearing impaired, or sensorily deprived. **D,** The best placement for the nurse when interviewing clients in wheelchairs, or even in conventional chairs if the client has better hearing in one ear than in the other. (From Burnside IM: *Nursing and the aged,* ed 3, St Louis, 1988, Mosby.)

To promote client comfort and sharing of data, the nurse and client should mutually establish the organization of the interview. The client should feel that the nurse is a caring person who treats others with respect. Self-esteem is enhanced if the client feels included in the decision-making process.

At the beginning of the interview, the nurse and client need to determine the most effective and comfortable distance and position for the session. The ability to see and hear within a comfortable territory is critical to the communication process (Figs. 2-1 to 2-3).

The appropriate use of touch during the interview can reduce the anxiety associated with the initial encounter. The importance of and comfort with touch is highly individual, but most older persons need and appreciate it. Burnside (1988) advises that the nurse does not have to be overly professional and cautious about the use of touch with the older adult client. However, a word of caution about the use of touch with the older adult—do not use touch in a condescending manner. Touch should always convey respect, car-

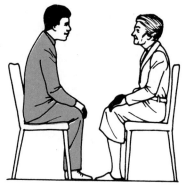

Fig. 2-2
Ordinarily the interviewer should sit very close to and facing an aged client. Sitting as close as 1 to 2 feet away is acceptable when there is loss of vision or hearing. If the individual seems guarded or frightened, the distance can be greater at the beginning of the interview and then lessened as the interview progresses. The interviewer should, of course, be seated, with head as near to the client's eye level as possible. (From Burnside IM: *Nursing and the aged,* ed 3, St Louis, 1988, Mosby.)

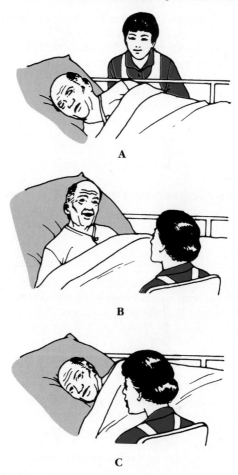

Fig. 2-3
Positions used with bedridden clients. **A,** An awkward, ineffective position to use with bedridden aged clients. **B,** A better position, but the nurse is still not close enough for frail, visually impaired, or hearing-impaired clients. **C,** The best position because the nurse is close to the client. (From Burnside IM: *Nursing and the aged,* ed 3, St Louis, 1988, Mosby.)

ing, and sensitivity. Do not be surprised if the older person reciprocates because of an unmet need for intimacy.

Finally, the nurse does not have to obtain the entire history in the traditional manner of a seated, face-to-face interview. In fact, this technique may be inappropriate with the older adult client, depending on the situation. The nurse should not overlook the natural opportunities available in the setting for gathering information. Interviewing the client during the bath, at mealtime, or even while participating in a game, hobby, or other social activity usually provides much more meaningful data.

The Client

Several factors influence the ability of the client to participate meaningfully in the interview. The nurse must be aware of these factors because they affect the older client's ability to communicate all of the information necessary for determining appropriate, comprehensive interventions. Sensory-perceptual deficits, anxiety, reduced energy level, pain, the multiplicity and interrelatedness of health problems, and the tendency to reminisce are the major client factors requiring special consideration while the nurse elicits the health history. Table 2-1 on pp. 21-22 contains recommendations for managing these factors.

Health History Format

The sample format for collecting a health history (see box on pp. 23-35) is an extensive one that focuses on the special needs and concerns of the older adult client. Although it may seem overwhelming and repetitive in places, remember that for this population there are many physical and psychosocial conditions that may be present, some of which may overlap. Depending on the setting and purpose, not every client will need to be asked every question. The suggested format can be used as a reference from which to proceed in collecting data from each client. The order of the components enables the nurse to begin with the less threatening, "get-acquainted" type of questioning that eases the tension and anxiety and builds trust. The nurse then gradually moves to the more personal and sensitive questions. If the client responds "yes" to any of the symptoms listed within the Review of Systems section of the sample health history tool, a full symptom analysis is necessary and will help guide the focus of the physical examination (Table 2-2).

Text continued on p. 35

Table 2-1   Client factors affecting history taking and recommendations

Factor	Recommendations
Visual disturbance	Position self in full view of client
	Provide diffuse, bright light; avoid glare
	Make sure client's glasses are worn and in good working order
	Face client when speaking; do not cover mouth
Hearing deficit	Speak directly to client in clear, low tones at a moderate rate; do not cover mouth
	Articulate consonants with special care
	Restate if client does not understand question initially
	Speak toward "good" ear
	Reduce background noises
	Make sure client's hearing aid is worn and is working properly
Anxiety	Give sufficient time to respond to questions
	Establish rapport and trust by acknowledging expressed concerns
	Determine mutual expectations of interview
	Use open-ended questions that indicate an interest in learning about the client
	Explain why information is needed
	Use a conversational style
	Allow for some degree of life review
	Offer a cup of coffee, tea, or soup
	Call the client by name often

Continued

Table 2-1   Client factors affecting history taking and recommendations—cont'd

Factor	Recommendations
Reduced energy level	Position comfortably to promote alertness
	Allow for more than one assessment encounter; vary the meeting times
	Be alert to subtle signs of fatigue: inability to concentrate, reduced attention span, restlessness, posture
Pain	Be patient; establish a slow pace for the interview
	Position comfortably to reduce pain
	Ask client about degree of pain; intervene before interview or reschedule
	Comfort and communicate through touch
	Use distraction techniques
	Provide a relaxed, "warm" environment
Multiplicity and interrelatedness of health problems	Be alert to subjective and objective cues about body systems and emotional and cognitive function
	Give client opportunity to prioritize physical and psychosocial health concerns
	Be supportive and reassuring about deficits created by multiple diseases
	Complete full analysis on all reported symptoms
	Be alert to reporting of new or changing symptoms
	Allow for more than one interview time
	Compare and validate data with old records, family, friends, or confidants
Tendency to reminisce	Structure reminiscence to gather necessary data
	Express interest and concern for issues raised by reminiscing
	Put memories into chronologic perspective to appreciate the significance and span of client's life

Table 2-2   Symptom analysis factors

Dimensions of a Symptom	Questions to Ask
1. Location	"Where do you feel it? Does it move around? Does it radiate? Show me where it hurts."
2. Quality or character	"What does it feel like?"
3. Quantity or severity	"On a scale of 1 to 10, with 10 being the worst pain you could have, how would you rate the discomfort you have now?"
	"How does this interfere with your usual activities?"
	"How bad is it?"
4. Timing	"When did you first notice it? How long does it last? How often does it happen?"
5. Setting	"Does this occur in a particular place or under certain circumstances? Is it associated with any specific activity?"
6. Aggravating or alleviating factors	"What makes it better? What makes it worse?"
7. Associated symptoms	"Have you noticed other changes that occur with this symptom?"

From Barkauskas VH et al: *Health and physical assessment,* ed 2, St Louis, 1998, Mosby.

HEALTH HISTORY FORMAT

1. Client Profile/Biographical Data
Name _____ Address _____
Telephone _____ Date and place of birth/age _____
Sex ___ Race ___ Religion _____ Marital status _____
Education _____ Nearest contact person _____
Address/Telephone _____

Continued

HEALTH HISTORY FORMAT—cont'd

2. Chief Complaint/Reason for Visit _____

_____

_____

_____

_____

3. Family Profile

Spouse(s)   Children
   Living _____   Living _____
   Health status _____   Names and addresses
   Age ____   _____
   Occupation _____   _____

   _____

   Deceased ____   Deceased ____
   Year of death _____   Year of death _____
   Cause of death _____   Cause of death _____

4. Occupational Profile

Current work status _____

Previous occupations _____

Source(s) of income and adequacy for needs _____

_____

_____

_____

5. Living Environment Profile

Type of dwelling _____

Number of rooms _____ Number of levels _____

Number of people living in dwelling _____

Degree of privacy _____ Nearest neighbor _____

Address/telephone _____

_____

6. Recreation/Leisure Profile

Hobbies/interests _____

Organizational memberships _____

Vacations/travel _____

7. Resources/Support Systems Used

Physician(s) _____

_____

Hospital _____

HEALTH HISTORY FORMAT—cont'd

Clinic _____

Home health agency _____

Meals on Wheels _____

Adult day care _____

Other _____

8. Description of Typical Day (type and amount of time spent in each activity; exercise patterns; problems/difficulties encountered with activities; usual bedtime ritual)

_____

_____

_____

9. Present Health Status

General health status during past year _____

_____

_____

General health status during past 5 years _____

_____

_____

Major health concerns _____

_____

Knowledge/understanding and management of health problems (e.g., special diet, dressing changes) _____

_____

_____

Overall degree of function relative to health problems and medical diagnoses _____

_____

Medications

Name(s) _____

_____

_____

Dosage _____

_____

How/when taken _____

_____

Continued

HEALTH HISTORY FORMAT—cont'd

Prescribing physician _____

Date of prescription _____

Problems with adherence (complicated regimen with large number and variety of drugs, visual deficits, unpleasant side effects, perception of effectiveness, difficulty obtaining, affordability)

Immunization status (note date of most recent immunization)

Tetanus, diphtheria _____

PPD _____

Influenza _____

Pneumovax _____

Allergies (note specific agent and reaction)

Drugs _____

Foods _____

Contact substances _____

Environmental factors _____

Nutrition

24-hour diet recall (include fluid intake)
Special diet, food restrictions, or preferences _____
_____
_____
History of weight gain/loss _____
Food consumption patterns (e.g., frequency, alone or with others) _____
_____
_____
Problems affecting food intake (e.g., inadequate income, lack of transportation, emotional stress) _____
_____
Habits _____
_____
_____

HEALTH HISTORY FORMAT—cont'd

10. Past Health Status
Childhood illnesses

_____

_____

_____

Serious or chronic illnesses

_____

_____

Trauma

_____

_____

Hospitalizations (note reason, date, place, duration, physician[s])

_____

_____

_____

Operations (note type, date, place, reason, physician[s])

_____

_____

_____

Obstetric history _____

_____

11. Family History
Draw genogram (identify grandparents, parents, aunts, uncles, siblings, spouse[s], children) (see p. 28 for sample)

Survey the following: cancer, diabetes mellitus, heart disease, hypertension, seizure disorder, renal disease, arthritis, alcoholism, mental health problems, anemia

12. Review of Systems
Check yes or no for each symptom and include full symptom analysis on positive responses at end of each system.

General	Yes	No
Fatigue		
Weight change in past year (note amount)		
Appetite change (note increase or decrease)		
Fever		

Continued

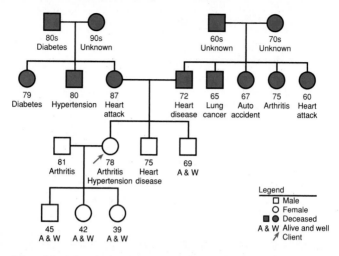

Adapted from Lueckenotte AG: *Gerontologic nursing,* St Louis, 1996, Mosby.

HEALTH HISTORY FORMAT—cont'd

General	Yes	No
Night sweats		
Sleeping difficulty		
Frequent colds, infections		
Self-rating of overall health status _____		
Ability to carry out ADLs _____		

Integument	Yes	No
Lesions/wounds		
Pruritus		
Pigmentation changes		
Texture changes		
Nevi changes		
Frequent bruising		
Hair changes		
Nail changes		
Corns, bunions, calluses		
Chronic sun exposure		
Healing pattern of lesions, bruises _____		

HEALTH HISTORY FORMAT—cont'd

Hematopoietic	Yes	No
Abnormal bleeding/bruising		
Lymph node swelling		
Anemia		
Blood transfusion history _____		

Head	Yes	No
Headache		
Past significant trauma		
Dizziness		
Scalp itching		

Eyes	Yes	No
Vision changes		
Glasses/contact lenses		
Pain		
Excessive tearing		
Pruritus		
Swelling around eyes		
Floaters		
Diplopia		
Blurring		
Photophobia		
Scotomata		
History of infections		
Date of most recent vision examination _____		
Date of most recent glaucoma check _____		
Impact on ADL performance _____		

Ears	Yes	No
Hearing changes		
Discharge		
Tinnitus		
Vertigo		
Hearing sensitivity		
Prosthetic device(s)		

Continued

HEALTH HISTORY FORMAT—cont'd

Ears	Yes	No
History of infection		
Date of most recent auditory examination _____		
Usual ear care habits _____		
Impact on ADL performance _____		

Nose and Sinuses	Yes	No
Rhinorrhea		
Discharge		
Epistaxis		
Obstruction		
Snoring		
Pain over sinuses		
Postnasal drip		
Allergies		
History of infections		
Self-rating of olfactory ability _____		

Mouth and Throat	Yes	No
Sore throat		
Lesions/ulcers		
Hoarseness		
Voice changes		
Difficulty swallowing		
Bleeding gums		
Caries		
Altered taste		
Difficulty chewing		
Prosthetic device(s)		
History of infections		
Date of most recent dental examination _____		
Brushing pattern _____		
Flossing pattern _____		
Denture cleaning routine and problems _____		

HEALTH HISTORY FORMAT—cont'd

Neck	Yes	No
Stiffness		
Pain/tenderness		
Lumps/masses		
Limited movement		

Breasts	Yes	No
Lumps/masses		
Pain/tenderness		
Swelling		
Nipple discharge		
Nipple changes		
Breast self-examination pattern _____		

Date and results of most recent mammogram _____

Respiratory	Yes	No
Cough		
Shortness of breath		
Hemoptysis		
Sputum		
Wheezing		
Asthma/respiratory allergy		
Date and results of most recent chest x-ray examination		

Cardiovascular	Yes	No
Chest pain/discomfort		
Palpitations		
Shortness of breath		
Dyspnea on exertion		
Paroxysmal nocturnal dyspnea		
Orthopnea		
Murmur		
Edema		
Varicosities		
Claudication		

Continued

HEALTH HISTORY FORMAT—cont'd

Cardiovascular	Yes	No
Paresthesias		
Leg color changes		

Gastrointestinal	Yes	No
Dysphagia		
Indigestion		
Heartburn		
Nausea/vomiting		
Hematemesis		
Appetite changes		
Food intolerances		
Ulcers		
Pain		
Jaundice		
Lumps/masses		
Change in bowel habits		
Diarrhea		
Constipation		
Melena		
Hemorrhoids		
Rectal bleeding		
Usual bowel pattern ———————————————		

Urinary	Yes	No
Dysuria		
Frequency		
Dribbling		
Hesitancy		
Urgency		
Hematuria		
Polyuria		
Oliguria		
Nocturia		
Incontinence		
Painful urination		
Stones		
Infections		

HEALTH HISTORY FORMAT—cont'd

Genitoreproductive—Male	Yes	No
Lesions		
Discharge		
Testicular pain		
Testicular mass(es)		
Prostate problems		
Venereal disease(s)		
Change in sex drive		
Impotence		
Concerns re: sexual activity		

Genitoreproductive—Female	Yes	No
Lesions		
Discharge		
Dyspareunia		
Postcoital bleeding		
Pelvic pain		
Cystocele/rectocele/prolapse		
Venereal disease(s)		
Infections		
Concerns re: sexual activity		

Menstrual history (age of onset, date of last menstrual period) _____

Menopausal history (age, symptoms, postmenopausal problems, use of hormone replacement therapy) _____

Date and result of most recent Pap test _____

Gr _____ P _____ A _____

Musculoskeletal	Yes	No
Joint pain		
Stiffness		
Joint swelling		
Deformity		
Spasm		
Cramping		
Muscle weakness		

Continued

HEALTH HISTORY FORMAT—cont'd

Musculoskeletal	Yes	No
Gait problems		
Back pain		
Prosthesis(es)		
Usual exercise pattern _____		
Impact on ADL performance		

Central Nervous System	Yes	No
Headache		
Seizures		
Syncope/drop attacks		
Paralysis		
Paresis		
Coordination problems		
Tic/tremor/spasm		
Paresthesias		
Head injury		
Memory problems		

Endocrine System	Yes	No
Heat intolerance		
Cold intolerance		
Goiter		
Skin pigmentation/texture changes		
Hair changes		
Polyphagia		
Polydipsia		
Polyuria		

Psychosocial	Yes	No
Anxious		
Depressed		
Insomnia		
Crying spells		
Nervous		
Fearful		

HEALTH HISTORY FORMAT—cont'd

	Psychosocial	Yes	No
Trouble with decision making			
Difficulty concentrating			
Statement of general feelings of satisfaction/frustration			
Usual coping mechanisms			
Current stresses			
Concerns about death			
Impact on ADL performance			

When assessing the older adult's use of medications, the nurse should recognize that drugs can cause problems with function, including cognition, mobility, continence, and balance. Also, certain drugs may be responsible for some symptoms the client may be reporting. Table 2-3 identifies the more commonly used/prescribed drugs in older adults and their effects. Be alert to the possibility of the older client's drugs producing undesirable effects and thus influencing symptom reporting.

Federal legislation (Omnibus Budget Reconciliation Act, 1987) mandates that nursing facilities providing nursing, medical, and rehabilitative care to Medicare or Medicaid beneficiaries conduct a comprehensive, standardized assessment of each resident's functional capacity, using a Resident Assessment Instrument (RAI) specified by the state. The key components of the RAI used in most states are the Minimum Data Set (MDS) and the Resident Assessment Protocols (RAPs). The MDS is the assessment and screening tool, while the RAPs identify triggers that may indicate potential problems. The RAPs also provide guidelines for follow-up assessment of potential problems. The MDS and RAP format is quite extensive, so it is not reproduced here. However, it is common in the long-term care setting, and its use reveals much about a resident's strengths, needs, and preferences.

Table 2-3   Drugs and their associated effects that can affect older adult assessment

Drug	Effect
Angiotensin-converting enzyme inhibitors (ACEIs)	Dry, nonproductive cough; taste disturbances
Antacids (magnesium or aluminum based)	Magnesium based: diarrhea; aluminum based: constipation
Anticholinergic agents Antihistamines Tricyclic antidepressants Cold remedies Antiparkinson agents Antipsychotic agents	Dry mouth; blurred vision; drowsiness; urinary retention; delirium; unsteady gait; falls; orthostatic hypotension; constipation
Anxiolytics	Sedation; impaired concentration; dizziness; unsteady gait; falls
Calcium channel antagonists	Constipation; peripheral edema; weight gain
Cardiovascular agents (reserpine, methyldopa, beta-blockers)	Depression
Corticosteroids	Depression; euphoria; gastrointestinal distress; insomnia
Histamine receptor antagonists (cimetidine)	Delirium
Hypnotics	"Hangover" effect; sedation; delirium; unsteady gait; falls
Narcotics	Depression; sedation; constipation
Nitrites/nitrates	Headache; flushing; dizziness
Nonsteroidal antiinflammatory drugs (NSAIDs) Corticosteroids Potassium Alcohol	Gastrointestinal distress
Salicylates	Tinnitus; vertigo; gastrointestinal distress

NOTE: This represents only a partial list of drugs having adverse effects that may affect assessment of the older adult client.

Functional, Cognitive, Affective, and Social Assessment

The traditional assessment, including the history, physical examination, and baseline laboratory data, does not by itself give the nurse the data necessary for planning nursing care. Standardized assessment tools to measure various aspects of functional and psychosocial status can be used as an adjunct to the traditional assessment. These assessments include observations of the older client's ability to perform activities of daily living (ADLs) and the client's cognitive, affective, and social functions. These additional data provide a more comprehensive view of the impact of all of the interrelated variables on the older client's total function.

Functional Status Assessment

Functional status assessment is a measurement of one's ability to perform ADLs independently. Determination of functional independence can identify client abilities and limitations, leading to the selection of appropriate interventions. The client situation determines the time of day when the test should be administered, as well as the number of times the client may need to be tested to ensure accurate results. Many tools are available, but the nurse should use only those that are valid, reliable, and relevant to the practice setting. The following is a description of tools that are appropriate for use with older adults in most settings.

The Katz Index of ADL (Katz et al, 1963) is a tool widely used to determine the results of treatment and the prognosis in the elderly and chronically ill (see box, pp. 38-40). The index ranks adequacy of performance in the six functions of bathing, dressing, toileting, transferring, continence, and feeding. A dichotomous rating of independence or dependence is made for each of the functions. Only people who can perform the function without any help at all are rated as independent; the actual evaluation form merely shows the rater how a dependent item is determined. The order of items reflects the natural progression in loss *and* restoration of function, based on studies conducted by Katz and his colleagues (Kane and Kane, 1981). It is a useful tool for the nurse because it describes the client's functional level at a specific point in time and objectively measures the effects of treatments intended to restore function. The tool only takes about 5 minutes to administer and can be used in most settings.

Katz Index of ADL

Index of Independence in Activities of Daily Living

The Index of Independence in Activities of Daily Living is based on an evaluation of the functional independence or dependence of patients in bathing, dressing, going to toilet, transferring, continence, and feeding. Specific definitions of functional independence and dependence appear below the index.

A—Independent in feeding, continence, transferring, going to toilet, dressing, and bathing

B—Independent in all but one of these functions

C—Independent in all but bathing and one additional function

D—Independent in all but bathing, dressing, and one additional function

E—Independent in all but bathing, dressing, going to toilet, and one additional function

F—Independent in all but bathing, dressing, going to toilet, transferring, and one additional function

G—Dependent in all six functions

Other—Dependent in at least two functions, but not classifiable as C, D, E, or F

Independence means without supervision, direction, or active personal assistance, except as specifically noted below. This is based on actual status and not on ability. A patient who refuses to perform a function is considered as not performing the function, even though he or she is deemed able.

Bathing (Sponge, Shower, or Tub)

Independent: assistance only in bathing a single part (such as back or disabled extremity) or bathes self completely

Dependent: assistance in bathing more than one part of body, assistance in getting in or out of tub, or does not bathe self

Dressing

Independent: gets clothes from closets and drawers; puts on clothes, outer garments, braces; manages fasteners; act of tying shoes is excluded

Dependent: does not dress self or remains partly undressed

Going to Toilet

Independent: gets to toilet; gets on and off toilet; arranges clothes; cleans organs of excretion (may manage own bedpan used at night only and may or may not be using mechanical supports)

Dependent: uses bedpan or commode or receives assistance in getting to and using toilet

Transfer

Independent: moves in and out of bed independently and moves in and out of chair independently (may or may not be using mechanical supports)

Dependent: assistance in moving in or out of bed and/or chair; does not perform one or more transfers

Continence

Independent: urination and defecation entirely self-controlled

Dependent: partial or total incontinence in urination or defecation; partial or total control by enemas, catheters, or regulated use of urinals and/or bedpans

Feeding

Independent: gets food from plate or its equivalent into mouth (precutting of meat and preparation of food, as buttering bread, are excluded from evaluation)

Dependent: assistance in act of feeding (see above); does not eat at all, or parenteral feeding

Evaluation Form

Name _____ Date of evaluation _____

For each area of functioning listed below, check the description that applies. (The word "assistance" means supervision, direction of personal assistance.)

Bathing—either sponge bath, tub bath, or shower

- Receives no assistance (gets in and out of tub by self if tub is usual means of bathing)
- Receives assistance in bathing only one part of the body (such as back or a leg)
- Receives assistance in bathing more than one part of the body (or not bathed)

Continued

Katz Index of ADL—cont'd

Dressing—gets clothes from closets and drawers (including underclothes, outer garments) and uses fasteners (including braces if worn)

- Gets clothes and gets completely dressed without assistance
- Gets clothes and gets dressed without assistance except for assistance in tying shoes
- Receives assistance in getting clothes or in getting dressed, or stays partly or completely undressed

Toileting—going to the "toilet room" for bowel and urine elimination; cleaning self after elimination, and arranging clothes

- Goes to "toilet room," cleans self, and arranges clothes without assistance (may use object for support such as cane, walker, or wheelchair and may manage night bedpan or commode, emptying same in morning)
- Receives assistance in going to "toilet room," in cleansing self, in arranging clothes after elimination, or in use of night bedpan or commode
- Doesn't go to "toilet room" for the elimination process

Transfer

- Moves in and out of bed as well as in and out of chair without assistance (may be using object for support such as cane or walker)
- Moves in or out of bed or chair with assistance
- Doesn't get out of bed

Continence

- Controls urination and bowel movement completely by self
- Has occasional "accidents"
- Supervision helps keep urine or bowel control; catheter is used, or is incontinent

Feeding

- Feeds self without assistance
- Feeds self except for getting assistance in cutting meat or buttering bread
- Receives assistance in feeding or is fed partly or completely by using tubes or intravenous fluids

From Katz S et al: Studies of illness in the aged. The index of ADL: a standardized measure of biological and psychological function, *JAMA* 185:94-99, 1963.

Cognitive/Affective Status Assessment

The multiple physiologic, psychologic, and environmental causes of cognitive impairment in older adults, coupled with the view that mental impairment is a normal, age-related process, often leads to incomplete assessment of this problem. Standardized examinations test a variety of cognitive functions, aiding identification of deficits that impact overall functional ability. Formal, systematic testing of mental status can help the nurse determine which behaviors are impaired and warrant interventions.

The Short Portable Mental Status Questionnaire (SPMSQ) (see the box on pp. 42-44), used to detect the presence and degree of intellectual impairment, consists of 10 items that test orientation, memory in relation to self-care ability, remote memory, and mathematical ability (Pfeiffer, 1975). The simple scoring method rates the level of intellectual functioning, which aids in making clinical decisions regarding self-care capacity.

The Mini-Mental State Exam (MMSE) (see the box on pp. 45-46) tests the cognitive aspects of mental functions: orientation, registration, attention and calculation, recall, and language (Folstein et al, 1975). The highest possible score is 30, with a score of 21 or less generally indicative of cognitive impairment requiring further investigation. The examination takes only a few minutes to complete and is easily scored, but it cannot be used alone for diagnostic purposes. Because the MMSE quantifies the severity of cognitive impairment and demonstrates cognitive changes over time and with treatment, it is a useful tool for assessing client progress in relation to interventions.

The Information-Memory-Concentration Test (IMCT) (Blessed et al, 1968), also called the Blessed Dementia Scale, is a test that quantifies changes in a client's: (1) ability to perform select aspects of everyday living tasks; (2) personality, interests, and drive; and (3) orientation, memory, and concentration. The Short Blessed Scale (SBT) is a revised version of the original IMCT, consisting of only six items (Katzman et al, 1983); it includes three orientation questions, the name and address memory phrase, counting from 20 to 1, and the months backward (see the box on p. 47). The tool is easily administered in a short period of time and reliably identifies clients with cognitive deficits. Katzman et al (1983) found the shortened version to highly correlate with neuropathologic findings of autopsied subjects ($p < .001$). It is considered to be more sensitive than the SPMSQ and the MMSE in detecting

Short Portable Mental Status Questionnaire (SPMSQ)

Instructions: Ask questions 1-10 in this list, and record all answers. Ask question 4A only if patient does not have a telephone. Record total number of errors based on ten questions.

+	−	
__	__	1. What is the date today? _____
		Month Day Year
__	__	2. What day of the week is it? _____
__	__	3. What is the name of this place? _____
__	__	4. What is your telephone number? _____
__	__	4A. What is your street address? _____
		(Ask only if patient does not have a telephone.)
__	__	5. How old are you? _____
__	__	6. When were you born? _____
__	__	7. Who is the President of the US now? __
__	__	8. Who was President just before him? __
__	__	9. What was your mother's maiden name? __
		10. Subtract 3 from 20 and keep subtracting 3 from each new number, all the way down.
	_____	Total number of errors

To Be Completed by Interviewer

Patient's name: _____ Date _____

Sex: __ Male   Race: __ White
     __ Female   __ Black
                           __ Other
Years of education: _____   __ Grade school
                              __ High school
                              __ Beyond high school

Interviewer's name: _____

Instructions for Completion of the Short Portable Mental Status Questionnaire (SPMSQ)

All responses to be scored as correct must be given by subject without reference to calendar, newspaper, birth certificate, or other aid to memory.

Short Portable Mental Status Questionnaire (SPMSQ)—cont'd

Question 1 is to be scored as correct only when the exact month, exact date, and the exact year are given correctly.

Question 2 is self-explanatory.

Question 3 should be scored as correct if any correct description of the location is given. "My home," correct name of the town or city of residence, or the name of hospital or institution if subject is institutionalized are all acceptable.

Question 4 should be scored as correct when the correct telephone number can be verified, or when the subject can repeat the same number at another point in the questioning.

Question 5 is scored as correct when stated age corresponds to date of birth.

Question 6 is to be scored as correct only when the month, exact date, and year are all given.

Question 7 requires only the last name of the President.

Question 8 requires only the last name of the previous President.

Question 9 does not need to be verified. It is scored as correct if a female first name plus a last name other than subject's last name is given.

Question 10 requires that the entire series must be performed correctly in order to be scored as correct. Any error in the series or unwillingness to attempt the series is scored as incorrect.

Scoring of the Short Portable Mental Status Questionnaire (SPMSQ)

The data suggest that both education and race influence performance on the Mental Status Questionnaire and they must accordingly be taken into account in evaluating the score attained by an individual.

For purposes of scoring, three educational levels have been established: *(a)* persons who have had only a grade school education; *(b)* persons who have had any high school education or who have completed high school; *(c)* persons who have had any education beyond the high school level, including college, graduate school, or business school.

Continued

Short Portable Mental Status Questionnaire (SPMSQ)—cont'd

For white subjects with at least some high school education, but not more than high school education, the following criteria have been established:

0-2 errors	Intact intellectual functioning
3-4 errors	Mild intellectual impairment
5-7 errors	Moderate intellectual impairment
8-10 errors	Severe intellectual impairment

Allow one more error if subject has had only a grade school education.

Allow one less error if subject has had education beyond high school.

Allow one more error for black subjects, using identical education criteria.

From Pfeiffer E: A short portable mental status questionnaire for the assessment of organic brain deficit in elderly patients, *J Am Geriatr Soc* 23:433-441, 1975.

Mini-Mental State Exam (MMSE)

Score

Maximum	Patient	

Orientation

| 5 | _____ | What is the (year) (season) (date) (day) (month)? |
| 5 | _____ | Where are we? (state) (county) (town) (hospital) (floor) |

Registration

| 3 | _____ | Name 3 objects: 1 second to say each. Then ask the patient all 3 after you have said them. Give 1 point for each correct answer. Then repeat them until he learns all 3. Count trials and record. Trials _____ |

Mini-Mental State Exam (MMSE)—cont'd

Attention and Calculation

5   _____   Serial 7s. 1 point for each correct. Stop after 5 answers. Alternatively spell "world" backwards.

Recall

3   _____   Ask for the 3 objects repeated above. Give 1 point for each correct.

Language

9   _____   Name a pencil and watch (2 points).
                     Repeat the following: "No ifs, ands, or buts" (1 point).
                     Follow a 3-stage command: "Take a paper in your right hand, fold it in half, and put it on the floor" (3 points).
                     Read and obey the following: "Close your eyes" (1 point).
                     Write a sentence (1 point).
                     Copy design (1 point).

Total score   _____

Assess level of consciousness along a continuum:

Alert   Drowsy   Stupor   Coma

Instructions for Administration of MMSE

Orientation

1. Ask for the date. Then ask specifically for parts omitted (e.g., "Can you also tell me what season it is?"). One point for each correct answer.
2. Ask in turn "Can you tell me the name of this hospital?" (town, county, etc.). One point for each correct answer.

Registration

Ask the client if you may test his or her memory. Then say the names of 3 unrelated objects, clearly and slowly, allowing about 1 second for each. After you have said all 3, ask him or her to repeat them. This first repetition determines his or her score (0-3) but keep saying them until he or she can repeat all 3, up to 6 trials. If he or she does not eventually learn all 3, recall cannot be meaningfully tested.

Continued

Mini-Mental State Exam (MMSE)—cont'd

Attention and calculation

Ask the patient to begin with 100 and count backward by 7. Stop after 5 subtractions (93, 86, 79, 72, 65). Score the total number of correct answers.

If the patient cannot or will not perform this task, ask him or her to spell the word "world" backward. The score is the number of letters in correct order (e.g., dlrow = 5, dlorw = 3).

Recall

Ask the patient if he or she can recall the 3 words you previously asked him or her to remember. Score 0-3.

Language

Naming: Show the patient a wrist watch and ask him or her what it is. Repeat for pencil. Score 0-2.

Repetition: Ask the patient to repeat the sentence after you. Allow only one trial. Score 0 or 1.

Three-stage command: Give the patient a piece of plain blank paper and repeat the command. Score 1 point for each part correctly executed.

Reading: On a blank piece of paper print the sentence "Close your eyes," in letters large enough for the patient to see clearly. Ask him to read it and do what it says. Score 1 point only if he actually closes his eyes.

Writing: Give the patient a blank piece of paper and ask him to write a sentence for you. Do not dictate a sentence, it is to be written spontaneously. It must contain a subject and verb and be sensible. Correct grammar and punctuation are not necessary.

Copying: On a clean piece of paper, draw intersecting pentagons, each side about 1 inch, and ask him to copy it exactly as it is. All 10 angles must be present and 2 must intersect to score 1 point. Tremor and rotation are ignored.

Estimate the patient's level of sensorium along a continuum, from alert on the left to coma on the right.

From Folstein MF, Folstein SE, McHugh PR: Mini-mental state: a practical method for grading the cognitive state of patients for the clinician, *J Psychiatr Res* 12:189-198, 1975.

Short Blessed Test

"Now I would like to ask you some questions to check your memory and concentration. Some of them may be easy and some of them may be hard."

	Maximum Error	Error Score	Weight	Weighted Score
1. What year is it now? _____	$\underline{1}$	_____	× 4 =	_____
2. What month is it now? _____	$\underline{1}$	_____	× 3 =	_____
Please repeat this phrase after me and remember it: John Brown, 42 Market Street, Chicago Number of trials to learning: _____				
3. About what time is it without looking at your watch (within 1 hour)? Response: _____ Actual time: _____	$\underline{1}$	_____	× 3 =	_____
4. Count backward from 20 to 1 (mark correctly sequenced numerals): 20 19 18 17 16 15 14 13 12 11 10 9 8 7 6 5 4 3 2 1	$\underline{2}$	_____	× 2 =	_____
5. Say the months of the year in reverse order (mark correct months): D N O S A JL JN MY AP M F J	$\underline{2}$	_____	× 2 =	_____
6. Repeat the name and address I asked you to remember John Brown 42 Market Street Chicago	$\underline{5}$	_____	× 2 =	_____
		Total Weighted Score		_____

Score ≥8 indicates impairment.

Name: _____   Date: _____

From Katzman R, et al: Validation of a short orientation-memory-concentration test of cognitive impairment, *Am J Psychiatry* 140:734-735, 1983.

early dementia because of the difficulty of reciting the months backward and the memory phrase questions. The usefulness of the test in distinguishing between demented and depressed older adults has not been determined.

Affective status measurement tools are used to differentiate the type of serious depression that affects function from the low mood common to many people. Depression is common in the elderly and frequently associated with confusion and disorientation, so depressed older persons are often mistakenly labeled *demented*. It is important to note here that people who are depressed usually respond to items on mental status examinations by saying "I don't know," which leads to poor performance. Since mental status examinations are not able to distinguish between dementia and depression, a response of "I don't know" should be interpreted as a sign that further affective assessment is warranted. Mental status examinations do not clearly distinguish between depression and dementia, so affective assessment is an important additional tool.

The Beck Depression Inventory (see the box on pp. 48-50) contains 13 items describing a variety of symptoms and attitudes associated with depression (Beck and Beck, 1972). Each item is rated using a 4-point scale to designate the intensity of the symptom. The tool is easily scored and can be self-administered or given by the nurse in about 5 minutes. Depending on the degree of impairment, the number of responses for each item could be confusing or could create difficulty for the older client. The nurse may need to assist clients experiencing this problem with the tool. The scoring cutoff points aid in estimating the severity of the depression (Beck and Beck, 1972).

The short form Geriatric Depression Scale (see the box on p. 52), distilled from the original 30-question Geriatric Depression Scale, is a convenient instrument designed specifically for use with older persons to screen for depression (Yesavage and Brink, 1983). Questions answered as indicated are scored 1 point. A score of 5 or more may indicate depression.

Social Assessment

The relationship the older adult has with family plays a central role in the overall level of health and well-being the older adult experiences. The assessment of this aspect of the client's social system can yield vital information about an important part of the total support network. Despite popular belief, families provide

Beck Depression Inventory, Short Form

Instructions: This is a questionnaire. On the questionnaire are groups of statements. Please read the entire group of statements in each category. Then pick out the one statement in that group which best describes the way you feel today, that is, *right now!* Circle the number beside the statement you have chosen. If several statements in the group seem to apply equally well, circle each one.

Be sure to read all the statements in each group before making your choice.

A. (Sadness)
  3 I am so sad or unhappy that I can't stand it.
  2 I am blue or sad all the time and I can't snap out of it.
  1 I feel sad or blue.
  0 I do not feel sad.

B. (Pessimism)
  3 I feel that the future is hopeless and that things cannot improve.
  2 I feel I have nothing to look forward to.
  1 I feel discouraged about the future.
  0 I am not particularly pessimistic or discouraged about the future.

C. (Sense of failure)
  3 I feel I am a complete failure as a person (parent, husband, wife).
  2 As I look back on my life, all I can see is a lot of failures.
  1 I feel I have failed more than the average person.
  0 I do not feel like a failure.

D. (Dissatisfaction)
  3 I am dissatisfied with everything.
  2 I don't get satisfaction out of anything anymore.
  1 I don't enjoy things the way I used to.
  0 I am not particularly dissatisfied.

E. (Guilt)
  3 I feel as though I am very bad or worthless.
  2 I feel quite guilty.
  1 I feel bad or unworthy a good part of the time.
  0 I don't feel particularly guilty.

Continued

Beck Depression Inventory, Short Form—cont'd

F. (Self-dislike)
  3 I hate myself.
  2 I am disgusted with myself.
  1 I am disappointed in myself.
  0 I don't feel disappointed in myself.

G. (Self-harm)
  3 I would kill myself if I had the chance.
  2 I have definite plans about committing suicide.
  1 I feel I would be better off dead.
  0 I don't have any thoughts of harming myself.

H. (Social withdrawal)
  3 I have lost all of my interest in other people and don't care about them at all.
  2 I have lost most of my interest in other people and have little feeling for them.
  1 I am less interested in other people than I used to be.
  0 I have not lost interest in other people.

I. (Indecisiveness)
  3 I can't make any decisions at all anymore.
  2 I have great difficulty in making decisions.
  1 I try to put off making decisions.
  0 I make decisions about as well as ever.

J. (Self-image change)
  3 I feel that I am ugly or repulsive-looking.
  2 I feel that there are permanent changes in my appearance and they make me look unattractive.
  1 I am worried that I am looking old or unattractive.
  0 I don't feel that I look any worse than I used to.

K. (Work difficulty)
  3 I can't do any work at all.
  2 I have to push myself very hard to do anything.
  1 It takes extra effort to get started at doing something.
  0 I can work about as well as before.

L. (Fatigability)
  3 I get too tired to do anything.
  2 I get tired from doing anything.
  1 I get tired more easily than I used to.
  0 I don't get any more tired than usual.

Beck Depression Inventory, Short Form—cont'd

M. (Anorexia)

3 I have no appetite at all anymore.

2 My appetite is much worse now.

1 My appetite is not as good as it used to be.

0 My appetite is no worse than usual.

Scoring

0-4   None or minimal depression

5-7   Mild depression

8-15   Moderate depression

16+   Severe depression

From Beck AT, Beck RW: Screening depressed patients in family practice: a rapid technique, *Postgrad Med* 52:81-85, 1972.

substantial help to their older members. Consequently, the level of family involvement and support cannot be disregarded when collecting data.

A short screening tool that can be used to assess the older person's social functioning is the Family APGAR (Smilkstein et al, 1982). Adaptation, partnership, growth, affection, and resolve (APGAR) are the aspects of family functioning that the tool assesses (see the box on p. 52-53). The tool can be easily adapted for use with clients who have more intimate social relationships with friends than family by simply substituting the term *friends* for *family* in the statements. A score of less than 3 suggests a highly dysfunctional family, with a score of 4 to 6 indicating a moderately dysfunctional family. The use of this screening instrument with a new client, or following a serious, stressful life event is appropriate.

The results of any of the tools just discussed for measuring functional and psychosocial status should be interpreted in view of all the data obtained from the client. A complete picture of the client can be determined only after careful analysis of all sources of data.

Yesavage Geriatric Depression Scale, Short Form

1. Are you basically satisfied with your life? (no)
2. Have you dropped many of your activities and interests? (yes)
3. Do you feel that your life is empty? (yes)
4. Do you often get bored? (yes)
5. Are you in good spirits most of the time? (no)
6. Are you afraid that something bad is going to happen to you? (yes)
7. Do you feel happy most of the time? (no)
8. Do you often feel helpless? (yes)
9. Do you prefer to stay home at night, rather than go out and do new things? (yes)
10. Do you feel that you have more problems with memory than most? (yes)
11. Do you think it is wonderful to be alive now? (no)
12. Do you feel pretty worthless the way you are now? (yes)
13. Do you feel full of energy? (no)
14. Do you feel that your situation is hopeless? (yes)
15. Do you think that most persons are better off than you are? (yes)

Score 1 point for each response that matches the yes or no answer after the question.

From Yesavage JA, Brink TL: Development and validation of a geriatric depression screening scale: a preliminary report, *J Psychiatr Res* 17:37-49, 1983.

Family APGAR

1. I am satisfied that I can turn to my family (friends) for help when something is troubling me. *(adaptation)*
2. I am satisfied with the way my family (friends) talks over things with me and shares problems with me. *(partnership)*
3. I am satisfied that my family (friends) accepts and supports my wishes to take on new activities or directions. *(growth)*

From Smilkstein G et al: Validity and reliability of the Family APGAR as a test of family function, *J Fam Pract* 15:303-311, 1982.

Family APGAR—cont'd

4. I am satisfied with the way my family (friends) expresses affection and responds to my emotions, such as anger, sorrow, or love. *(affection)*
5. I am satisfied with the way my friends and I share time together. *(resolve)*

Scoring:

Statements are answered *always* (2 points), *some of the time* (1 point), *hardly ever* (0 points).

References

Barkauskas VH et al: *Health and physical assessment,* ed 2, St Louis, 1998, Mosby.

Beck AT, Beck RW: Screening depressed patients in family practice: a rapid technique, *Postgrad Med* 52:81-85, 1972.

Blessed G, Tomlinson B, Roth M: The association between quantitative measures of dementia and senile change in cerebral grey matter in the elderly, *Br J Psychiatry* 114:797-811, 1968.

Burnside IM: *Nursing and the aged: a self-care approach,* ed 3, St Louis, 1988, Mosby.

Folstein MF, Folstein SE, McHugh PR: Mini-mental state: a practical method for grading the cognitive state of patients for the clinician, *J Psychiatr Res* 12:189-198, 1975.

Kane RA, Kane RL: *Assessing the elderly: a practical guide to measurement,* Lexington, MA, 1981, Lexington Books.

Katz S et al: Studies of illness in the aged. The index of ADL: a standardized measure of biological and psychological function, *JAMA* 185:94-99, 1963.

Katzman R et al: Validation of a short orientation-memory-concentration test of cognitive impairment, *Am J Psychiatry* 140:734-739, 1983.

Pfeiffer E: A short portable mental status questionnaire for the assessment of organic brain deficit in elderly patients, *J Am Geriatr Soc* 23:433-441, 1975.

Smilkstein G et al: Validity and reliability of the Family APGAR as a test of family function, *J Fam Pract* 15:303-311, 1982.

Yesavage JA, Brink TL: Development and validation of a geriatric depression screening scale: a preliminary report, *J Psychiatr Res* 17:37-49, 1983.

Physical
Assessment

3

Approach and Overview

Examination Approach and Sequence

The objective information acquired in the physical examination adds to the subjective data base already gathered. Together, these components serve as the basis for establishing nursing diagnoses, planning, developing interventions, and evaluating nursing care.

Physical examination is typically performed after the health history. The approach should be a systematic and deliberate one that allows the nurse to (1) determine client strengths and capabilities as well as disabilities and limitations, (2) gain objective support for subjective data, and (3) gather objective data not previously known.

There is no single right way to put together the parts of the physical examination, but a head-to-toe approach is generally the most efficient. The sequence used to conduct the physical examination within this approach is an individual one, depending on the individual older adult client. In all cases, however, a side-to-side comparison of findings is made using the client as the control. To promote mastery in conducting an integrated and comprehensive physical examination, the nurse should develop a method of organization and use it consistently.

Ultimately, the practice setting and client condition together determine the type and method of examination to be performed. For example, a client admitted to an acute care hospital with a medical diagnosis of congestive heart failure will initially require respiratory and cardiovascular system assessments to plan interventions for improving activity tolerance. In the home care setting, assessment of the client's musculoskeletal system is a priority for determining fall-related injury potential and ability to perform basic self-care tasks. The frail, immobile client in a long-term care setting will require an initial skin assessment to determine risk for pressure ulcer development and preventive measures required. Frequent, regular examination of the skin thereafter is necessary to assess effectiveness of the prevention measures instituted.

In all of the above situations, complete physical examinations are important and should eventually be carried out, but client and setting dictate priorities. Consider the subjective client data already obtained in terms of the urgency of the situation, the acute or chronic nature of the problem, the extent of the problem on the basis of body systems affected, and the interrelatedness of physical and psychosocial factors in determining where to begin.

General Guidelines

Regardless of the approach and sequence used, the following principles should be kept in mind while conducting the physical examination:

- Be alert to the older client's energy level. If the situation warrants it, complete the examination at another time. Generally, it should take approximately 30 to 45 minutes to conduct the examination.
- Respect the client's modesty. Allow privacy for changing into a gown; if assistance is needed, do so in such a way so as not to expose the client's body or cause embarrassment. Keep the client comfortably draped; do not unnecessarily expose a body part.
- Sequence the examination to keep position changes to a minimum. Clients with limited range of motion and strength may require assistance. Be prepared to use alternative positions if the client is unable to assume the usual position for examination of a body part.
- Develop an efficient sequence for examination that minimizes both nurse and client movement. Variations that may be necessary will not be disruptive if the sequence is followed consistently. Working from one side of the patient, generally the right side, promotes efficiency.
- Ensure comfort for the client. Offer a blanket for added warmth and a pillow for comfortable positioning.
- Explain each step in simple, clear terms. Warn of any discomfort that might occur. Be gentle.

- Share findings with the client to reassure when possible. Encourage client to ask questions.
- Project warmth, sincerity, and interest in client.
- Develop a standard format on which to note selected findings. Not all data must be recorded; try to reduce the potential for forgetting certain data, particularly measurements.

Equipment for Physical Examination

Because the older adult client may become easily fatigued during the physical examination, the nurse should ensure proper functioning and readiness of all equipment before the examination begins to avoid unnecessary delays. Place the equipment within easy reach and in the order in which it will be used (see the box on p. 57).

Physical Examination Skills

Inspection

Inspection is the deliberate use of the eyes and nose to gather data. Learn to observe the client during the initial encounter to gain valuable clues that can influence the remainder of the assessment. For example, as the client enters the room, note the general appearance, posture, and gait. While shaking hands with introductions, note grip, mobility, eye contact, speech, breathing pattern, skin color, and dress. These quick but careful observations can reveal clues about the client's musculoskeletal and neurologic system integrity, mental and emotional status, and interest in and ability to provide self-care.

Inspection continues throughout the interview and physical assessment. The following guidelines should be considered:

- Adequate lighting and exposure are essential to careful inspection of color, size, texture, and mobility.
- Tangential lighting may be necessary for noting the contour of and variations in the body surface.
- As each body part is examined, note symmetry with the opposite side of the body.
- Observe unhurriedly, pay attention to detail, and record findings.
- Watch carefully how the client follows instructions and carries out maneuvers to obtain data regarding functional ability.

Equipment for Physical Examination

Sphygmomanometer
Stethoscope with diaphragm and bell
Thermometer
Tuning fork with frequencies of 500 to 1000 cps
Otoscope
Ear and nasal specula
Ophthalmoscope
Percussion hammer
Penlight
Measuring tape (180 to 200 cm)
10 cm transparent, flexible pocket ruler
Sharp and dull testing implements
Marking pen
Tongue depressors
Cerumen spoon
Olfactory testing substances
Taste testing substances
Examination gloves
Cotton-tipped applicators
Cotton balls
Lubricant
Visual acuity screening chart
Scale with height measurement rod
Tissues

Specimen Gathering Materials

Culture media
Occult blood testing materials
Vaginal speculum (Pederson)
Pap smear spatula
Sterile cotton-tipped applicator
Glass slides
Fixative

Detection of odors as part of inspection is important when examining older adults. Foul body odors may be a result of poor hygiene or disease. Strong perfume and cologne odors may indicate a diminished sense of smell. Such a finding should alert the nurse to a potential safety hazard if the client would be unable to detect the odor of gas or smoke.

Palpation

Palpation is the use of the hands and fingers to gather data through touch. The characteristics of body texture, temperature, size, shape, and movement are distinguished by different parts of the hands and fingers. The fingertips are most sensitive to touch, with sensitivity enhanced by using a slightly circular motion. The palm and ulnar surfaces are used for distinguishing vibrations, and the dorsal surface is best for estimating temperature.

Warm hands and short fingernails are essential in avoiding client discomfort. The client should be in a relaxed position as gentle but deliberate palpation is carried out. Any known areas of tenderness are palpated last.

Since sensitivity to touch can be dulled by continuous and heavy pressure on the fingertips, the nurse should use light palpation initially. If findings so indicate, one may progress to deep palpation. Deep palpation is always necessary to examine abdominal contents, but exerting pressure with the sensing hand diminishes its sensitivity. The fingers of the dominant hand are placed on the area to be palpated, then the fingers of the other hand are placed immediately on top of and slightly behind the first set of fingers. Pressure is exerted with the top fingers while the first set of fingers palpates.

A bimanual technique uses both hands to entrap an organ or mass between the fingertips to better assess its size and shape. Ballottement is another technique of palpation used to evaluate organ consistency or fluid tension with a bouncing or tapping motion of the fingertips. Pressure is exerted by one fingertip while another, sensing fingertip assesses the impact. This technique is carried out in rapid sequence.

Age-specific variations of palpation with the older adult are as follows:

- Since tactile sensation dulls with age, a deeper palpation is necessary to elicit a response when assessing sensations of sharp/dull, light/deep, hot/cold, and tenderness.
- Declines in vision, hearing, and touch require that instructions be given clearly and distinctly to ensure adequate understanding.
- Decreased muscle mass, tone, strength, endurance, and agility; calcification of cartilage and ligaments; and a decreased bone mass are variables that can make limb and joint palpation painful and tiring. Be alert to signs of discomfort and fatigue, and alter the examination as needed.

- Loss of skin elasticity and increased wrinkling require assessment of turgor on the abdomen.
- Arterial wall thickening and loss of elasticity result in absent or decreased pulses on palpation.

Percussion

Percussion is used to assess the size, position, and density of underlying structures. The technique consists of a sharp tapping that produces vibrations and subsequent sound waves. The sound waves are heard as percussed tones. Percussion is an aid to assessing the presence of air, fluid, and solid material in an underlying structure.

The direct method of percussion is carried out by striking the body surface directly with one or two partially bent fingers. The indirect method, the most widely used, is performed by placing the distal phalanx of the middle finger (pleximeter) of the nondominant hand flat against the area to be percussed. The percussion blow is struck by the tip of the middle finger of the dominant hand. The target of the blow is the interphalangeal joint of the pleximeter finger, or the area just distal to that joint. The blow is delivered by movement of only the wrist; the forearm remains stationary. The blow should be sharp and rapid, snapping the wrist back quickly. The fingernail must be short. Repeated practice of this technique is necessary to acquire the skill.

The sounds produced by percussion are classified according to the acoustical properties of the tones produced, from loudest to softest (Table 3-1). Alterations in tonal quality as a result of age are also noted.

Auscultation

Auscultation is the process of listening to sounds produced by the organs and tissues of the body. It is a clinical tool used most frequently to assess the heart, lungs, neck, and abdomen. The complexity of the sounds and the difficulty in distinguishing normal from abnormal require practice listening to the normal sounds. Only when the nurse becomes experienced in recognizing normal sounds can abnormal sounds be confidently detected.

Sounds are characterized according to pitch, intensity, quality, and duration. Pitch is a measure of waves per second; more waves produce higher frequency and pitch. Intensity is a measure of the amplitude of the sound waves produced and ranges from high (loud sound) to low (soft sound). Quality is a property of sound

Table 3-1   Percussion sounds and properties

Percussion Sound	Intensity/Quality	Pitch	Sample Location	Age-Related Variations
Tympany	Loud, drumlike	High musical quality	Gastric air bubble, bowel	Sound will vary depending on bowel contents (dull to flat)
Hyperresonance	Loud, booming	Very low	Emphysematous lung	Hyperresonance in very thin, older client
Resonance	Loud, hollow	Low	Normal lung	
Dullness	Medium, thudlike	High	Liver	
Flatness	Soft, dull	High	Thigh	

Modified from Bates B: *A guide to physical examination and history taking*, ed 5, Philadelphia, 1991, JB Lippincott.

determined by its overtones; it is what distinguishes a particular sound from others of the same pitch and intensity. Duration is a measure of the length of time a sound lasts. The auscultation of any sound requires an assessment of these characteristics so a determination of normal or abnormal can be made.

Auscultation must be conducted in a quiet environment. Concentration is critical to accurate identification of sounds and their characteristics. Closing one's eyes can help in focusing on and isolating individual sounds. The nurse must fully assess each sound before moving systematically to the others. The diaphragm of the stethoscope is used to listen to high-pitched tones, the bell for detecting low-pitched tones.

Reference

Bates B: *A guide to physical examination and history taking,* ed 5, Philadelphia, 1991, JB Lippincott.

Nutritional Assessment

4

Older adults experience a wide variety of nutritional problems and needs related to the physical, socioeconomic, and environmental changes associated with aging. In fact, a substantial number of older adults are at high risk of poor nutritional status, including deficiency, dehydration, undernutrition, and obesity. Risk factors for poor nutritional status commonly occurring in this age group include the presence of acute or chronic diseases and conditions, inadequate or inappropriate food intake, inadequate financial resources, functional dependence or disability, and medications.

The components of nutritional status assessment include anthropometric measurement, biochemical measurement, clinical examination, and dietary analysis. The various applications of each of these four components are listed in Table 4-1. Although these components have been historically recognized as the standard by which nutritional assessment is conducted, there are special challenges with older adults.

What is known about the intricate relationships between nutrition and aging is continuously evolving. In some cases, references indicating the nutritional status of older adults have not even been established, making the interpretation of assessment data difficult. In addition, some of the physiologic changes associated with aging are hard to differentiate from clinical signs of nutrient deficiencies. Finally, data collected that may indicate a nutritional problem may also result from nonnutritional causes (Kuczmarski and Kuczmarski, 1993).

Nutrition plays a key role in disease prevention, health promotion, management of chronic health problems, and treatment of acute illness and injury. Although the approach to nutritional care is typically one that includes the team of nurse, physician, and di-

Table 4-1   Nutritional assessment methods and their purpose

Method	Purpose
Anthropometric	Determine and monitor body weight to detect changes in weight
	Determine and monitor body composition, especially body fat and water
	Determine body fat distribution to assess risk for selected chronic conditions
Biochemical	Determine and monitor nutritional risk for selected chronic conditions such as heart disease
	Determine and monitor the level of recent dietary intakes of selected nutrients
	Determine and monitor nutrient stores
	Obtain functional measures of nutritional adequacy or deficiency
	Confirm or refute nutritional diagnoses based on other assessment measures
	Determine immune function
Clinical	Determine presence of signs or symptoms diagnostic of nutritional deficiency or toxicity
	Determine and monitor ability to perform ADLs
	Evaluate and monitor dental health
	Evaluate cognitive status
	Determine whether signs or symptoms indicative of nutritional problems are reversed by nutritional intervention
Dietary	Obtain actual food and beverage intakes to determine quality of diet
	Monitor food consumption patterns of individuals or groups to identify changes and trends over time
	Determine usage of supplements and their effect on nutrient intake
	Evaluate feeding practices of institutionalized older adults

From Kuczmarski MF, Kuczmarski RJ: Nutritional assessment of older adults. In Schlenker ED: *Nutrition in aging,* ed 2, St Louis, 1993, Mosby.

etitian, the nurse usually performs the initial assessment or screening. Consequently, the nurse plays a key role in detecting actual or potential nutritional problems and making the appropriate referrals to the dietitian and/or physician.

Nutrition Screening

Nutrition screening is the process of identifying those characteristics known to be associated with dietary or nutritional problems for the purposes of differentiating those who are at high risk of nutritional problems or who have poor nutritional status. Screening may reveal the need for more in-depth analysis or assessment, providing additional information for diagnosis, treatment, and counseling.

Early detection of risk factors known to be associated with nutrition-related conditions can delay or prevent the onset of diseases and their subsequent complications. As a result, interventions can be put in place that may reduce the number and degree of functional impairments and disabilities, improve the quality of life, and even reduce the morbidity and mortality associated with disease, outcomes that are also correlated with decreased health care costs. The box on p. 65 categorizes risk factors associated with poor nutritional status in older adults and includes select elements by which risk is assessed. The greater the number of these risk factors, and the longer they persist, the greater is the probability that poor nutritional status will develop (Nutrition Screening Initiative, 1994).

The American Academy of Family Physicians, the American Dietetic Association, and the National Council on the Aging formed the Nutrition Screening Initiative in 1990 in response to the growing belief that nutritional status is indeed a "vital sign." The Determine Your Nutritional Health Checklist (see box, pp. 66-67) is a public awareness tool that can be self-administered and scored, or used by a caregiver. The checklist describes in simple language the warning signs of poor nutritional status and serves as a baseline for further nutritional assessment and intervention for identified problems.

The checklist consists of two parts: (1) a self-assessment protocol, which includes a series of statements that help people recognize aspects of their eating habits and life-style that places them at nutritional risk, and (2) DETERMINE, a mnemonic device that

Risk Factors Associated With Poor Nutritional Status in Older Americans, Including Elements by Which Risk is Assessed

Inappropriate Food Intake

Meal/snack frequency
Quantity/quality
  Milk/milk products
  Meat/meat substitutes
  Fruit/vegetables
  Bread/cereals
  Fats
  Sweets
Dietary modifications
  Self-imposed
  Prescribed
  Compliance
  Impact
Alcohol abuse

Poverty

Low income
  Source
  Adequacy
Food expenditures/
  resources
Economic assistance pro-
  gram reliance
  Food
  Housing
  Medical
  Other
  Adequacy

Social Isolation

Support systems
  Availability
  Utilization
Living arrangements
  Cooking/food storage
  Transportation
  Other

Dependency/Disability

Functional status
  Activities of daily living
    (ADLs)
  Instrumental activities of
    daily living (IADLs)
Disabling conditions
  Lack of manual dexterity
  Use of assistive devices
Inactivity/immobility

Acute/Chronic Disease or Conditions

Abnormalities of body
  weight
Alcohol use
Cognitive or emotional im-
  pairment
  Depression
  Dementias
Oral health problems
Pressure sores/ulcers
Sensory impairment
Others

Chronic Medications Use

Prescribed/self-
  administered
Polypharmacy
Nutritional supplements
Quackery

Advanced Age

From *Incorporating nutrition screening and interventions into medical practice: a monograph for physicians,* Washington, D.C., 1994, The Nutrition Screening Initiative.

Nutrition Screening Initiative Checklist

The warning signs of poor nutritional health are often overlooked. Use this checklist to find out if you or someone you know is a risk.

Read the statements below. Circle the number in the yes column for those that apply to you or someone you know. For each yes answer, score the number in the box. Total your nutritional score.

Determine Your Nutritional Health

	YES
I have an illness or condition that made me change the kind and/or amount of food I eat.	2
I eat fewer than 2 meals per day.	3
I eat few fruits or vegetables, or milk products.	2
I have 3 or more drinks of beer, liquor or wine almost every day.	2
I have tooth or mouth problems that make it hard for me to eat.	2
I don't always have enough money to buy the food I need.	4
I eat alone most of the time.	1
I take 3 or more different prescribed or over-the-counter drugs a day.	1
Without wanting to, I have lost or gained 10 pounds in the last 6 months.	2
I am not always physically able to shop, cook and/or feed myself.	2
TOTAL	

Total Your Nutritional Score. If it's –

0-2 Good! Recheck your nutritional score in 6 months

3-5 You are at moderate nutritional risk.
See what can be done to improve your eating habits and lifestyle. Your office on aging, senior nutrition program, senior citizens center or health department can help. Recheck your nutritional score in 3 months.

6
or more **You are at high nutritional risk.**
Bring this checklist the next time you see your doctor, dietitian or other qualified health or social service professional. Talk with them about any problems you may have. Ask for help to improve your nutritional health.

These materials developed and distributed by the Nutrition Screening Initiative, a project of:

AMERICAN ACADEMY OF FAMILY PHYSICIANS

THE AMERICAN DIETETIC ASSOCIATION

NATIONAL COUNCIL ON THE AGING

Sponsored in part through a grant from Ross Products Division, Abbott Laboratories.

Remember that warning signs suggest risk, but do not represent diagnosis of any condition. Turn the page to learn more about the Warnings Signs of poor nutritional health.

provides education about nutritional risk factors and indicators. The higher the score, the lower is the level of nutrient intake when compared with the Recommended Dietary Allowances. Although not a diagnostic tool, the checklist is a valid and reliable measure of potential nutrition risk, while at the same time educating people about risk factors.

Nutrition Screening Initiative Checklist—cont'd

The Nutrition Checklist is based on the Warning Signs described below. Use the word DETERMINE to remind you of the Warning Signs.

Disease
Any disease, illness or chronic condition which causes you to change the way you eat, or makes it hard for you to eat, puts your nutritional health at risk. Four out of five adults have chronic diseases that are affected by diet. Confusion or memory loss that keeps getting worse is estimated to affect one out of five or more of older adults. This can make it hard to remember what, when or if you've eaten. Feeling sad or depressed, which happens to about one in eight older adults, can cause big changes in appetite, digestion, energy level, weight and well-being.

Eating Poorly
Eating too little and eating too much both lead to poor health. Eating the same foods day after day or not eating fruit, vegetables, and milk products daily will also cause poor nutritional health. One in five adults skip meals daily. Only 13% of adults eat the minimum amount of fruit and vegetables needed. One in four older adults drink too much alcohol. Many health problems become worse if you drink more than one or two alcoholic beverages per day.

Tooth Loss/Mouth Pain
A healthy mouth, teeth and gums are needed to eat. Missing, loose or rotten teeth or dentures which don't fit well or cause mouth sores make it hard to eat.

Economic Hardship
As many as 40% of older Americans have incomes of less that $6,000 per year. Having less—or choosing to spend less—than $25-30 per week for food makes it very hard to get the foods you need to stay healthy.

Reduced Social Contact
One-third of all older people live alone. Being with people daily has a positive effect on morale, well-being and eating.

Multiple Medicines
Many older American must take medicines for health problems. Almost half of older Americans take multiple medicines daily. Growing old may change the way we respond to drugs. The more medicines you take, the greater the chance for side effects such as increased or decreased appetite, change in taste, constipation, weakness, drowsiness, diarrhea, nausea, and others. Vitamins or minerals when taken in large doses act like drugs and can cause harm. Alert your doctor to everything you take.

Involuntary Weight Loss/Gain
Losing or gaining a lot of weight when you are not trying to do so is an important warning sign that must not be ignored. Being overweight or underweight also increases your chance of poor health.

Needs Assistance in Self Care
Although most older people are able to eat, one of every five have trouble walking, shopping, buying and cooking food, especially as they get older.

Elder Years Above Age 80
Most older people lead full and productive lives. But as age increases, risk of frailty and health problems increase. Checking your nutritional health regularly makes good sense.

The Nutrition Screening Initiative, 1010 Wisconsin Avenue, NW, Suite 800, Washington, D.C. 20007
The Nutrition Screening Initiative is funded in part by a grant from Ross Laboratories, a division of Abbott Laboratories.

Anthropometric Measurement

Anthropometric measurement is the measurement of stature, body weight, composition, and proportions and is the foundation of nutritional assessment of older adults. When measurements are taken and recorded at regular intervals, they can provide a picture of nutritional status over time, thus allowing for quick identification of nutritional problems before the onset of serious health consequences.

Biochemical Measurement

There are a number of biochemical measures used to determine alterations in nutritional status. Biochemical measures in general are more sensitive than anthropometric methods in reflecting such alterations; when a nutrient deficiency occurs, tissue stores are depleted and the resulting reduction in the reserve stores and body fluids, metabolic products, and nutrient-dependent enzyme activity become detectable.

The following list of biochemical measures indicative of nutritional status is intended to serve as a guideline; each client situation should be viewed individually for the appropriateness or necessity of conducting the measurements. The reader is referred to a nutrition text for further information regarding biochemical indicators for specific nutrient deficiencies.

Serum albumin   Serum transferrin
Total iron binding capacity   Hemoglobin/hematocrit
Total lymphocyte count   Electrolytes
Cholesterol   Triglycerides
High density lipoproteins (HDL)   Low density lipoproteins (LDL)
LDL:HDL ratio   Serum folate
Serum vitamin B_{12}

Clinical Examination

Clinical examination includes the data obtained during the physical examination. The nurse should be alert to the observable signs indicating nutritional deficiencies or overnutrition. Assessment of functional status, particularly the IADLs, cognitive status, and the condition of the oral cavity, should be given special attention. Table 4-2 on pp. 69-74 identifies physical signs of nutritional diseases.

Dietary Analysis

A number of methods exist for obtaining information related to a client's dietary intake and patterns. The 24-hour recall is the easiest and fastest way to obtain data related to food intake, but it may be misleading or inadequate, since it only provides a

Text continued on p. 75

Table 4-2 Clinical signs and possible nutrient deficiency in adults

Clinical Signs	Consider Deficiency	Definition/Comment
Hair		
Easily pluckable, sparse	Protein, biotin	
Straight, dull	Protein	
Coiled, corkscrewlike	Protein	
	Vitamin A, vitamin C	Caused by follicular and keratinization change
Skin		
Xerosis	Essential fatty acid	Dryness of skin/aging, loss of skin lubricants
Petechiae	Vitamin A, vitamin C	Pin-head sized hemorrhages
Pigmentation	Niacin	Sign of pellagra distributed symmetrically in sun-exposed areas; also seen in hemochromatosis
Follicular keratosis	Vitamin A, possibly essential fatty acid	Keratin plugs in follicles, "goose flesh"
"Flaky-paint" dermatitis	Protein	
Subcutaneous fat loss, fine wrinkling	Protein-energy	Aging process
Poor tissue turgor	Water	Aging process

Adapted from Heymsfield SB, Williams PJ: Nutritional assessment by clinical and biochemical methods. In *Modern nutrition in health and disease*, ed 7, Philadelphia, 1988, Lea & Febiger.

Continued

Table 4-2 Clinical signs and possible nutrient deficiency in adults—cont'd

Clinical Signs	Consider Deficiency	Definition/Comment
Skin—cont'd		
Edema	Protein, thiamin	Seen in protein-energy malnutrition with hypoalbuminemia and in wet beriberi resulting from thiamin deficiency
Purpura	Vitamin C, vitamin K	Also seen in vitamin E toxicity
Perifollicular hemorrhage	Vitamin C	
Pallor	Folacin, iron, vitamin B_{12}, copper, biotin	
Tendency toward excessive bruising (ecchymoses)	Vitamin C, vitamin K	Caused by increased fragility of capillary walls; aging process
Pressure sores	Protein-energy	
Seborrheic dermatitis	Essential fatty acid, pyridoxine, zinc, biotin	
Poor wound healing	Protein-energy, zinc, and possibly essential fatty acids	
Thickening of skin	Essential fatty acid	
Eyes		
Dull, dry (xerosis) conjunctiva	Vitamin A	Can lead to xerophthalmia in severe deficiency
Keratomalacia	Vitamin A	Softening of cornea

		Early evidence of deficiency
Bitot's spot	Vitamin A	
Corneal vascularization	Riboflavin	
Photophobia	Zinc	
Lips and Oral Structures		
Angular fissures, scars, or stomatitis	B-complex, iron, protein, riboflavin	Also seen with ill-fitting dentures
Cheilosis	B₆, niacin, riboflavin, protein	Also seen with ill-fitting dentures, exposure to sun or cold
Ageusia, dysgeusia	Zinc	Also associated with altered sense of smell
Swollen, spongy, bleeding gums	Ascorbic acid	If not edentulous
Tongue		
Magenta tongue	Riboflavin	
Fissuring, raw	Niacin	
Glossitis	Pyridoxine, folacin, iron, vitamin B₁₂	Also seen with food irritants, antibiotic administration, uremia
Fiery red tongue	Folacin, vitamin B₁₂	Seen if anemia is not pronounced
Pale	Iron, vitamin B₁₂	Seen in severe cases
Atrophic papillae	Riboflavin, niacin, iron	Also seen with ill-fitting dentures, food irritants, aging

Continued

Table 4-2   Clinical signs and possible nutrient deficiency in adults—cont'd

Clinical Signs	Consider Deficiency	Definition/Comment
Nails		
Spoon-shaped nails (koilonychia)	Chromium, iron	
Brittle, ridged, lined nails	Nonspecific	May be protein undernutrition
Heart		
Tachycardia, cardiomegaly, congestive heart failure	Thiamin	"Wet" beriberi associated with high output congestive heart failure
Decreased cardiac function	Phosphorus	
Cardiac arrhythmias	Magnesium, potassium	
Small heart, decreased output, bradycardia	Protein-energy	Prone to congestive heart failure during refeeding
Abdomen		
Hepatomegaly	Protein	Fatty liver/commonly seen in alcoholics
Wasting	Energy	Found in marasmus
Enlarged spleen	Iron	Found in 15% to 25% of subjects with a significant degree of iron deficiency anemia
Bones		
Bone pain	Calcium, vitamin D, phosphorus, vitamin C	Seen in osteomalacia

Muscles, extremities		
Wasting	Protein-energy	
Pain in calves, weak thighs	Thiamin	
Edema	Protein, thiamin	Also seen with sodium toxicity and hypertension
Muscular twitching	Pyridoxine	
Muscular pains	Biotin, selenium	
Muscular weakness	Sodium, potassium	
Muscle cramps	Sodium, chloride	
Neurologic		
Ophthalmoplegia, footdrop	Thiamin	Wernicke's encephalopathy
Disorientation	Thiamin, sodium, water	Korsakoff's psychosis; fabrication occurs in thiamin-deficient alcoholics
Decreased position, vibratory sense, ataxia, optic neuritis	Vitamin B_{12}	Subacute spinal cord degeneration
Weakness, paresthesia of legs (burning and tingling)	Thiamin, pyridoxine, pantothenic acid, vitamin B_{12}	Nutritional polyneuropathy, especially with alcoholism; "burning foot" syndrome with pantothenic acid deficiency
Hyporeflexia	Thiamin	Aging process
Mental disorders	Niacin, magnesium, vitamin B_{12}	In untreated B_{12} deficiency, mental disorders may progress to severe psychosis

Continued

Table 4-2   Clinical signs and possible nutrient deficiency in adults—cont'd

Clinical Signs	Consider Deficiency	Definition/Comment
Neurologic—cont'd		
Convulsions	Pyridoxine, calcium, magnesium, phosphorus	
Depression, lethargy	Biotin, folacin, vitamin C	Aging process
Sleep disturbances	Pantothenic acid	Aging process
Peripheral neuropathy	Pyridoxine	
Other		
Diarrhea	Niacin, folacin, vitamin B_{12}	Also seen in vitamin C toxicity
Delayed wound healing and tissue repair	Vitamin C, zinc, protein-energy	
Anemia, pallor	Vitamin E, pyridoxine, vitamin B_{12}, iron, folacin, biotin, copper	
Anorexia	Vitamin B_{12}, chloride, sodium, thiamin, vitamin C	Also seen with vitamin A, zinc, or iron toxicity
Nausea	Biotin, pantothenic acid	
Fatigue, lassitude, apathy	Energy, biotin, pantothenic acid, magnesium, phosphorus, iron, potassium, sodium	

1-day account of foods eaten. With this method, the client is instructed to recall everything consumed during the previous 24 hours, including all foods, fluids, and supplements; include the time foods are eaten and amounts consumed, as well as any between-meal snacks.

Another method involves having the client keep a food diary or log for a designated number of days, usually 1 to 5. In addition to having the client record the date and time of food intake and the foods and fluids consumed, it may be beneficial to include the place where food is eaten, whether or not the client ate alone or with others, and the mood while eating. Caregivers or family members may need to assist the older adult client who has impairments that prevent gathering the data independently.

Once the data are obtained, the food records are analyzed to determine the client's actual intake of an adequate diet. Controversy exists as to whether or not the RDAs, based on age and sex, are applicable to older adults, since they represent average nutrient allowances for healthy people. Food intake patterns and practices can be evaluated against the Food Guide Pyramid (Fig. 4-1, p. 86), which outlines the types and amounts of foods to eat on a daily basis. The actual number of servings one should consume depends on energy needs. Eating the fewest number of servings for each of the food groups provides approximately 1600 kcal, which may be appropriate for some older adults. Eating the midpoint range of servings for each of the major food groups provides about 2200 kcal; the highest number of servings consumed provides about 2800 kcal (Kuczmarski and Kuczmarski, 1993).

Anthropometric Assessment

Equipment needed:

> Measuring stick or nonstretchable tape attached to a flat,
> vertical surface
> Some form of a right-angle headboard
> Standing platform scale
> Skinfold caliper
> Sliding broad-blade caliper*
> Measuring tape

*Anthropometric caliper (device to measure knee height) available from MediForm
Printers and Publishers, 5150 SW Griffith Drive, Beaverton, OR 97005.

Step

Measure Height

Technique: Minimum clothing should be worn so that posture
can be seen clearly. Ask client to stand up straight, with bare
heels close together, legs straight, arms at sides, shoulders
relaxed. Lower headboard onto the crown of the head. Have
client take a deep breath. Take measurement at point of
maximum inspiration with your eyes at headboard level to
avoid errors. Record measurement to nearest 0.1 cm or ½
inch.

	Normal/Individual Variations/Deviations		
Percentiles for stature in cm (and inches)			
Men			
Age (years)	95%	50%	5%
65	181.6 (71.5)	170.3 (67.0)	159.1 (62.6)
70	181.6 (71.5)	169.9 (66.9)	158.7 (62.5)
75	181.2 (71.3)	169.5 (66.7)	158.4 (62.4)
80	180.9 (71.2)	169.1 (66.6)	158.0 (62.2)
85	180.5 (71.1)	168.8 (66.5)	157.7 (62.1)
90	180.2 (70.9)	168.5 (66.3)	157.3 (61.9)
Women			
Age (years)	95%	50%	5%
65	171.6 (67.6)	161.0 (63.4)	153.1 (60.3)
70	169.8 (66.9)	159.1 (62.6)	151.3 (59.6)
75	167.9 (66.1)	157.3 (61.9)	149.4 (58.8)
80	166.1 (65.4)	155.4 (61.2)	147.6 (58.1)
85	164.2 (64.6)	153.6 (60.5)	145.7 (57.4)
90	162.4 (63.9)	151.7 (59.7)	143.9 (56.6)

From *Nutritional assessment of the elderly through anthropometry,* Columbus, OH, 1988, Ross Laboratories.

DEVIATIONS: A discrepancy between client's perception of height and the actual measurement

Continued

Step

Measure Weight

Technique: Calibrate scale to zero. Weigh before breakfast if possible, after bladder has been emptied, nude or in light clothing, without shoes. Position feet over center of platform. Adjust weights on balance beam, then read and record measurement at nearest 0.1 kg or ¼ lb.

Normal/Individual Variations/Deviations

Percentiles for weight in kg (and lb)

Men

Age (years)	95%	50%	5%
65	102.0 (224.9)	79.5 (175.0)	62.6 (138.0)
70	99.1 (218.5)	76.5 (168.7)	59.7 (131.6)
75	96.3 (212.3)	73.6 (162.3)	56.8 (125.2)
80	93.4 (205.9)	70.7 (155.9)	53.9 (118.8)
85	90.5 (199.5)	67.8 (149.5)	51.0 (112.4)
90	87.6 (193.1)	64.9 (142.8)	48.1 (106.0)

Women

Age (years)	95%	50%	5%
65	87.1 (192.0)	66.8 (147.3)	51.2 (112.9)
70	84.9 (187.2)	64.6 (142.4)	49.0 (108.0)
75	82.8 (182.5)	62.4 (137.6)	46.8 (103.2)
80	80.6 (177.7)	60.2 (132.7)	44.7 (98.5)
85	78.4 (172.8)	58.0 (127.9)	42.5 (93.7)
90	76.2 (168.0)	55.9 (123.2)	40.3 (88.8)

From *Nutritional assessment of the elderly through anthropometry,* Columbus, OH, 1988, Ross Laboratories.

DEVIATIONS: A discrepancy between client's perception of weight and the actual measurement; recent gain or loss; sudden increase of up to 5 lb per day may indicate fluid retention; >20% over IBW indicates obesity

Continued

Step

Knee height (to estimate stature of a client who cannot stand)

Technique: Have client lie supine with left knee and ankle each
bent at 90-degree angle. Place fixed blade of caliper under
heel of left foot. Place movable blade on top of thigh, at least
2 inches behind kneecap. From side of calf, make sure shaft
of caliper passes over anklebone and just behind head of
fibula. Hold shaft of caliper parallel to shaft of lower leg.
Apply pressure to compress tissue, and take measurement;
record to nearest 0.1 cm. Repeated measurements should
agree within 0.5 cm.

Stature can be estimated from knee height measurement using
the following formula:

$$\text{Men} = [2.02 \times \text{Knee height}] - [0.04 \times \text{Age}] + 64.19$$

$$\text{Women} = [1.83 \times \text{Knee height}] - [0.24 \times \text{Age}] + 84.88$$

If the knee height has been recorded in inches, it must be multi-
plied by 2.54 to convert to cm.

Midarm circumference (MAC)

Technique: With client's nondominant arm relaxed and bent at a
90-degree angle, with the forearm placed palm down across
the middle of the body, measure circumference at midpoint of
arm between tip of acromial process of scapula and olecranon
process of ulna. Record to estimate muscle wasting.

Normal/Individual
Variations/Deviations

Mid-upper arm circumference for older males and females by race

Age (years)	Percentile		
	5th (cm)	50th (cm)	95th (cm)
White			
Males			
55-64	27.5	32.3	37.6
65-74	25.5	31.6	36.8
Females			
55-64	25.1	30.8	39.4
65-74	24.3	30.5	38.8
Black			
Males			
55-64	27.2	32.6	39.6
65-74	24.6	30.6	38.2
Females			
55-64	25.5	33.5	45.1
65-74	26.1	32.7	39.1

Modified from Najjar MF, Rowland M: *Anthropometric reference data and prevalence of overweight, United States, 1976-1980,* Vital and Health Statistics, Series 11, No 238, DHHS Publication No (PHS) 87-1688, Washington, DC, 1987, US Government Printing Office.

Continued

Step

Triceps skinfold thickness (TSF)

Technique: Have client lie on right side with right arm extending from front of body. Position trunk in straight line, legs slightly tucked up. Position left arm along trunk, palm down. Grasp double fold of skin and subcutaneous fat tissue between fingers and thumb at level of midpoint marked for MAC. Fold is picked up on back of arm parallel to length of arm and just to right or left of level of midpoint mark, depending on which is easier for measurer. Place jaws of caliper perpendicular to length of skinfold at level of midpoint mark. Exert force with index finger and thumb until lines on caliper are aligned. After about 3 seconds, read measurement to nearest 2 mm. Repeated measurements should agree within 4 mm.

Normal/Individual
Variations/Deviations

Triceps skinfold for older males and females by race

Age (years)	Percentile		
	5th (mm)	50th (mm)	95th (mm)
White			
Males			
55-64	5.5	12.0	24.5
65-74	5.0	12.0	25.0
Females			
55-64	12.5	26.0	43.1
65-74	12.0	25.0	41.1
Black			
Males			
55-64	3.5	10.5	29.0
65-74	4.0	10.0	27.5
Females			
55-64	12.0	28.5	46.0
65-74	11.5	29.0	47.5

Modified from Najjar MF, Rowland M: *Anthropometric reference data and prevalence of overweight, United States, 1976-1980,* Vital and Health Statistics, Series 11, No 238, DHHS Publication No (PHS) 87-1688, Washington, DC, 1987, US Government Printing Office.

Continued

	Step	

Triceps skinfold thickness (TSF)—cont'd

Estimate body muscle mass using the following formula:

$$\text{Midarm muscle area} = \frac{\left[\text{MAC} - \left(3.14 \times \dfrac{\text{TSF}}{10}\right)\right]^2}{12.56}$$

Normal/Individual
Variations/Deviations

Percentiles for midarm muscle area in cm^2

Age (years)	Men		
	95%	50%	5%
65	77.1	59.4	43.2
70	75.3	57.7	41.4
75	73.5	55.9	39.6
80	71.7	54.1	37.8
85	69.9	52.3	36.0
90	68.2	50.5	34.3

Age (years)	Women		
	95%	50%	5%
65	66.4	44.5	33.5
70	65.9	44.1	33.0
75	65.5	43.6	32.6
80	65.1	43.2	32.2
85	64.7	42.8	31.8
90	64.2	42.4	31.3

From *Nutritional assessment of the elderly through anthropometry,* Columbus, OH, 1988, Ross Laboratories.

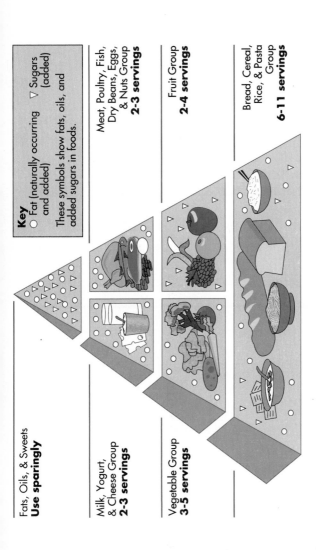

Fig. 4-1
Food Guide Pyramid. (From Human Nutrition Information Service: *USDA's food guide pyramid, Home and Garden Bull 249,* Hyattsville, MD, 1992, US Department of Agriculture.)

References

Heymsfield SB, Williams PJ: Nutritional assessment by clinical and biochemical methods. In Shils ME, Young VR, editors: *Modern nutrition in health and disease,* ed 7, Philadelphia, 1988, Lea & Febiger.

Human Nutrition Information Service: *USDA's food guide pyramid, Home and Garden Bull 249,* Hyattsville, MD, 1992, US Department of Agriculture.

Incorporating nutrition screening and interventions into medical practice: a monograph for physicians, Washington, D.C., 1994, The Nutrition Screening Initiative.

Kuczmarski MF, Kuczmarski RJ: Nutritional assessment of older adults. In Schlenker ED: *Nutrition in aging,* ed 2, St Louis, 1993, Mosby.

Najjar MF, Rowland M: *Anthropometric reference data and prevalence of overweight, United States, 1976-80,* Vital and Health Statistics, Series 11, No 238, DHHS Publication No (PHS) 87-1688, Washingtion, DC, 1987, US Government Printing Office.

Nutritional assessment of the elderly through anthropometry, Columbus, OH, 1988, Ross Laboratories.

General Survey and Mental Status Assessment

5

The general survey begins during the initial nurse-client encounter. Concentrated and unobtrusive inspection by the nurse of the client walking into the room, meeting the nurse, and following brief instructions provides an overall impression of the client's general state of health. These observations are not related to any particular body system or systems but reflect a quick and careful head-to-toe scan of the client. The components of this introductory survey are chronologic age versus apparent age, sex, race, body development, grooming and hygiene, facial expressions, and speech. The written descriptions of these introductory findings should be concise.

The purpose of mental status or cerebral function assessment is to determine the thoughts and mental processes that interfere with the older adult's attainment of optimal level of functioning. An essential component of this assessment is identification of the onset and historical progression of symptoms and behaviors. Interviewing collateral sources is usually indicated if abnormalities are suspected or obvious.

Mental status assessment is integrated into the interview and physical examination. Evaluate the client's awareness and orientation, cognitive abilities, mood, and affect. Observe physical appearance, behavior, and responses to questions. Test the components of the examination (see pp. 89-93) in a natural, nonthreatening manner with consideration of ethnicity. Proceed to

Text continued on p. 93

General Assessment

NOTE: Only inspection is used for this assessment.

Step	Normal Findings/Individual Variations/Deviations
Inspect client and client's means of negotiating the environment as client enters the room	Maneuvers safely and purposefully within setting DEVIATIONS: Aimless wandering, hesitation, drawing back, or aggressive posture and movement
Introduce self and offer to shake hands	Client establishes eye contact; facial expression appropriate to conversation; introduces self, and extends hand DEVIATIONS: Client does not establish eye contact, withdraws body from greeting; does not regard examiner with facial expression, speech, or handshake
Position self at eye level with client and explain purpose of encounter	Client listens attentively and acknowledges communication with nods, short comments, and phrases; asks questions for clarification DEVIATIONS: Facial expression exhibits anxiety, pain, apathy, hostility, fear; easily distracted
Observe skin (particularly face), hair, and speed and freedom of bodily movements to get clues for estimating apparent age	Creases, wrinkles, and frown lines; graying, dry, or brittle hair Reduced speed and coordination; use of ambulatory aids; small, shuffling steps with stooped posture

Continued

Step	Normal Findings/Individual Variations/Deviations
	DEVIATIONS: Marked wrinkling of skin; no scalp or body hair, excessive thinning of hair; hirsutism; foot dragging, limping, or shuffling; tremor, contracture; asymmetric movement; rigid posture
Inspect body development	Height and weight within acceptable norms for age; symmetric size and shape of body parts
	Slight carrying angle deformities in elbow, knee, wrist, fingers, or neck; muscles and tendons more prominent
	Fat redistribution from extremities to trunk
	DEVIATIONS: Excessively tall or short; asymmetric size and/or shape of parts; excessive muscle wasting; loss of muscle or muscle group; obesity or cachectic appearance
Note grooming/hygiene	Hair clean, combed
	Nails clean and trimmed; may be dull and brittle
	Clothing clean and appropriate
	No odors
	DEVIATIONS: Hair uncombed and dirty; dirty, ragged nails; dirty, unkempt clothing; inappropriate, bizarre dress combinations; foul body odors; fetid breath, fruity odor, ammonia-like odor
Observe facial expression	Makes eye contact; smiles, and shows thoughtful, reflective expressions appropriate to conversation

Step	Normal Findings/Individual Variations/Deviations
	Symmetric facial features DEVIATIONS: No eye contact; motionless face, fixed stare; eyes darting around, lip licking or biting, hiding mouth behind hand when speaking or smiling (tension, fear); grimacing (pain); pale, perspiring, or tearful; asymmetric features as evidenced by paralysis, contracture, muscle atrophy, and flattening
Note speech: Comprehension	Follows simple instructions, answers questions DEVIATIONS: Difficulty responding to questions and instructions; circumlocution and perseveration; evasive replies
Articulation	Enunciates clearly Overall moderate pace with variations appropriate to topic DEVIATIONS: Difficulty articulating a specific speech sound; rapid-fire delivery, hesitancy, stuttering, repetitions, or slow, monotonous speech
Note mental status: Orientation	Oriented to person, place, and time as evidenced by history

Continued

Step	Normal Findings/Individual Variations/Deviations
	DEVIATIONS: Unable to give accurate, current biographical data (name, address, birthdate); unable to identify year, season, date (NOTE: If unable to recall date, determine what cues are normally present in client's environment to promote orientation before labeling abnormal.)
Attention and concentration	Relates history in clear, logical manner and answers questions directly without drifting from subject (NOTE: Reminiscence is normal.) Regards examiner appropriately during interaction
	DEVIATIONS: Decreased or slowed thinking (depression); wandering off of subject; irrelevant responses; fragmented, incoherent, illogical thought processes (delirium); decreased attention (fatigue, anxiety, or medication related)
Judgment	Responses during interview indicate ability to manage personal, interpersonal, and social aspects of life
	DEVIATIONS: Unable to evaluate a situation and determine appropriate reaction

Step	Normal Findings/Individual Variations/Deviations
Memory	*Remote:* Accurate recall of past medical history (NOTE: Interviewer must have access to correct answers from collateral sources.)
	DEVIATIONS: Unable to recall data, events; confabulation
	Recent: Accurate recall of remembrances after several minutes to an hour; some hesitation
	DEVIATIONS: Unable to recall data, events
Thought content and processes	Rational, logical, and realistic thinking; relates history in a clear, sequential, and logical manner
	DEVIATIONS: Delusional content; loosening of associations; incoherent, illogical; flight of ideas
Mood and affect	Stable and sustained mood during interview; mild anxiety
	Appropriate fluctuations of affect according to subject being discussed
	DEVIATIONS: Labile mood; apprehensive, fearful, sense of dread; blunted, flat, or inappropriate affect

one of the standardized mental examinations discussed in Chapter 2 for more extensive assessment when abnormalities are detected. However, be cautious in administering these tools, for they do not take into account sensory deficits, culture, and life-style of the older adult.

Describe mental status assessment findings in simple, direct terms. Avoid words with many connotations, such as "preoccupied," "suspicious," or "hostile." Document the client's behaviors and statements objectively, accurately, and succinctly to reduce the potential for broad interpretation.

Regardless of the setting in which the initial encounter takes place, be alert to the older client's need to take more time to acclimate to the surroundings and purpose of the assessment. Adjust pace, offer reassurance, and project honesty, warmth, and interest as the client is assisted in getting settled.

Assessment of Integument

6

The skin, or integument, and its associated structures of glands, hair, and nails constitute the integumentary system. The assessment of integument is usually integrated throughout the physical examination as each of the other systems is assessed. The skills of inspection, palpation, and mensuration are used. A transparent pocket ruler and penlight are the only equipment needed.

Skin lesions should be described in terms of type (Tables 6-1 and 6-2), size, color, distribution, and configuration. Distribution refers to the location or body region affected and the symmetry of findings in comparable body parts. Configuration refers to the arrangement of lesions in relation to each other.

The following terms are commonly used to describe the configuration of skin lesions:

Arciform	Bow-shaped
Annular	Circle, ring-shaped
Confluent	Merged together
Grouped	Clustered together
Herpetiform or zosteriform	Clustered vesicles erupting unilaterally along the course of cutaneous nerves
Linear	Line arrangement
Polycyclic	Multiple annular lesions

Anatomy and Physiology

The integument consists of three main layers: epidermis, dermis, and hypodermis (Fig. 6-1). The epidermis is the superficial outer layer, made up primarily of keratinocytes. Keratin is a protein that toughens and waterproofs the skin. Melanocytes, which synthesize

Text continued on p. 103

Table 6-1   Primary skin lesions (initial spontaneous manifestations of underlying pathological process)

Lesion	Description
Macule	Flat, nonpalpable, circumscribed; less than 1 cm in diameter; brown, red, purple, white, or tan in color (e.g., freckles, flat moles, rubella, rubeola)

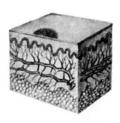

Patch	Flat, nonpalpable, irregularly shaped macule that is greater than 1 cm in diameter (e.g., vitiligo, port-wine marks)

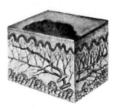

Papule	Elevated, palpable, firm, circumscribed; less than 1 cm in diameter; brown, red, pink, tan, or bluish red in color (e.g., warts, drug-related eruptions, pigmented nevi)

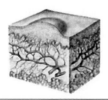

Table 6-1   Primary skin lesions (initial spontaneous manifestations of underlying pathological process)—cont'd

Lesion	Description
Plaque	Elevated, flat-topped, firm, rough, superficial papule greater than 1 cm in diameter; may be coalesced papules (e.g., psoriasis, seborrheic and actinic keratoses)

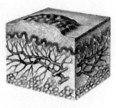

Wheal	Elevated, irregular-shaped area of cutaneous edema; solid, transient, changing; variable diameter; pale pink in color (e.g., urticaria, insect bites)

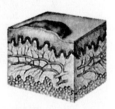

Nodule	Elevated, firm, circumscribed, palpable; deeper in dermis than papule; 1 to 2 cm in diameter (e.g., erythema nodosum, lipomas)

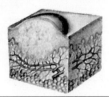

Continued

Table 6-1 Primary skin lesions (initial spontaneous
manifestations of underlying pathological process)—cont'd

Lesion	Description
Tumor	Elevated, solid; may or may not be clearly demarcated; greater than 2 cm in diameter; may or may not vary from skin color (e.g., neoplasms)

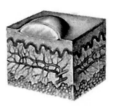

Vesicle	Elevated, circumscribed, superficial; filled with serous fluid; less than 1 cm in diameter (e.g., blister, varicella)

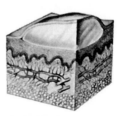

Bulla	Vesicle greater than 1 cm in diameter (e.g., blister, pemphigus vulgaris)

Table 6-1   Primary skin lesions (initial spontaneous manifestations of underlying pathological process)—cont'd

Lesion	Description
Pustule	Elevated, superficial; similar to vesicle but filled with purulent fluid (e.g., impetigo, acne, herpes zoster)

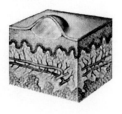

| Cyst | Elevated, circumscribed, palpable, encapsulated; filled with liquid or semisolid material (e.g., sebaceous cyst) |

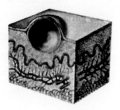

| Telangiectasia | Fine, irregular red line produced by dilation of capillary (e.g., telangiectasia in rosacea) |

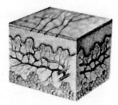

From Thompson JM: *Clinical outlines for health assessment,* St Louis, 1997, Mosby.

Table 6-2   Secondary skin lesions (later evolution of a primary lesion or external trauma to the primary lesion)

Lesion	Description
Scale	Heaped-up keratinized cells; flaky exfoliation; irregular; thick or thin; dry or oily; varied size; silver, white, or tan in color (e.g., psoriasis, exfoliative dermatitis)

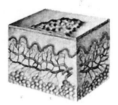

Crust	Dried serum, blood, or purulent exudate; slightly elevated; size varies; brown, red, black, tan, or straw in color (e.g., scab on abrasion, eczema)

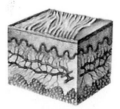

Lichenification	Rough, thickened epidermis, accentuated skin markings resulting from rubbing or irritation, often involves flexor aspect of extremity (e.g., chronic dermatitis)

Table 6-2   Secondary skin lesions (later evolution of a primary lesion or external trauma to the primary lesion)—cont'd

Lesion	Description
Scar	Thin to thick fibrous tissue replacing injured dermis; irregular; pink, red, or white in color; may be atrophic or hypertrophic (e.g., healed wound or surgical incision)

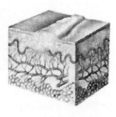

Lesion	Description
Keloid	Irregularly shaped, elevated, progressively enlarging scar; grows beyond boundaries of wound; caused by excessive collagen formation during healing (e.g., keloid from ear piercing or burn scar)

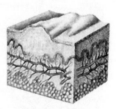

Lesion	Description
Excoriation	Loss of epidermis; linear or hollowed-out crusted area, dermis exposed (e.g., abrasion, scratch)

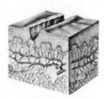

Continued

Table 6-2   Secondary skin lesions (later evolution of a primary lesion or external trauma to the primary lesion)—cont'd

Lesion	Description
Fissure	Linear crack or break from epidermis to dermis; small, deep, red (e.g., athlete's foot, cheilois)

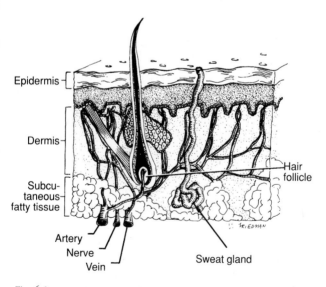

From Thompson JM: *Clinical outlines for health assessment,* St Louis, 1997, Mosby.

Fig. 6-1
Cross-section of the skin reveals three layers: epidermis, dermis, and subcutaneous fatty tissue. (From Potter PA: *Pocket guide to health assessment,* ed 3, St Louis, 1994, Mosby.)

melanin and give skin its color, are also located in the epidermis. Melanin protects the body against the damaging effects of ultra-violet rays in sunlight. The main function of the epidermis is to protect the body from trauma, bacterial invasion, and drying.

In old age, the epidermis is thin and flattened, which is particularly obvious over bony prominences, forearms, lower legs, and the dorsal surface of hands and feet. This thinning causes veins to appear more prominent. Although melanin remains in keratinocytes, the number of functioning melanocytes decreases, thus increasing the keratinocyte-melanocyte ratio. Abnormal proliferation of the remaining melanocytes occurs, resulting in senile lentigines, a spotty pigmentation on the sun-exposed areas of the body, usually the dorsal surface of the hands and forearms. Various other surface skin lesions commonly occur in older persons (Table 6-3).

Table 6-3   Commonly occurring normal skin lesions in older people

Skin Lesion	Description
Seborrheic keratosis	Pigmented (light tan to black) macular-papular lesion seen on neck, chest, back, and at the hair line; can be warty, scaly, or greasy in appearance
Senile ectasias (senile or cherry angioma)	Bright, ruby-red or purplish papular lesions, 1 to 5 mm in size, found on trunk, upper chest, and extremities
Acrochordons (cutaneous skin tags)	Soft, pinkish tan to light brown pedunculated lesions on neck, upper chest, and axillary folds
Senile lentigines	Gray-brown, irregular, macular lesions on sun-exposed areas of the face, arms, and hands
Sebaceous hyperplasia	Yellowish, slightly elevated; with time becomes dome-shaped and umbilicated; found on forehead, lower lid, nose, and cheeks

The dermis is the thick connective tissue layer consisting of collagen, elastic, and reticulin fibers that provides support to the skin. The dermis is highly vascular, and it contains sensory nerve endings, hair follicles, eccrine glands, apocrine (sweat) glands, and sebaceous (oil) glands. Temperature regulation is also partially controlled by the dermis through blood vessel and apocrine gland activity.

Less collagen is formed in aging, and there is a decreased amount of elastic fiber, resulting in a more wrinkled appearance. The texture of the skin is drier because of fewer eccrine glands and decreased activity of both eccrine and sebaceous glands. The overall degeneration of the connective tissue, coupled with a decrease in total body water, contributes to decreased skin turgor.

The deepest layer of the skin is the hypodermis, or subcutaneous layer, where fat is manufactured and stored. This layer also insulates and cushions the body and regulates temperature.

Because of redistribution of body fat with aging, and general loss of elasticity with years of gravitational pull, the skin of the

Table 6-4   Systemic disorders associated with pruritus in the elderly

System	Disorder
Renal	Chronic renal failure
Hepatic	Extrahepatic biliary obstruction
	Hepatitis
	Drug ingestion
Hematopoietic	Polycythemia vera
	Hodgkin's disease
	Other lymphomas and leukemias
	Multiple myeloma
	Iron deficiency anemia
Endocrine	Hyperthyroidism
	Diabetes mellitus
Miscellaneous	Visceral malignancies
	Opiate ingestion
	Drug ingestion
	Psychosis

From Gilchrest BA: Skin diseases in the elderly. In Calkins E et al, eds: *The practice of geriatrics,* Philadelphia, 1986, Saunders, p 493.

older adult sags on the bony frame. The appearance of facial jowls, a double chin, and drooping beneath the eyes and earlobes is more obvious.

Older persons frequently experience localized or generalized pruritus that can be a mild nuisance or that can lead to extensive, slowly healing ulcers. Several systemic disorders are often associated with pruritus in the elderly (Table 6-4).

Pressure ulcers are a common clinical problem of the older adult population. The primary cause is chronic unrelieved pressure, resulting in tissue ischemia and eventually necrosis. Appendix D details the prediction and prevention of pressure ulcers. A

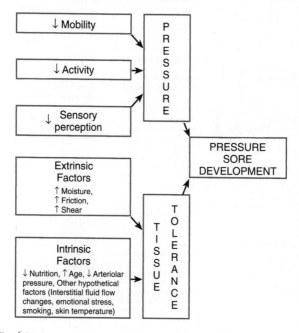

Fig. 6-2
Conceptual schema for the etiology of pressure sores. (Redrawn from Braden B, Bergstrom B: A conceptual schema for the study of the etiology of pressure sores, *Rehab Nurs* 12[1]:9, 1987. Copyright © 1987 by the Association of Rehabilitation Nurses. Reprinted with permission.)

Patient's Name _____   Evaluator's Name _____

SENSORY PERCEPTION (ability to respond meaningfully to pressure-related discomfort)	**1. Completely limited:** Unresponsive (does not moan, flinch, or grasp) to painful stimuli, due to diminished level of consciousness or sedation. **or** limited ability to feel pain over most of body surface.	**2. Very Limited:** Responds only to painful stimuli. Cannot communicate discomfort except by moaning or restlessness. **or** has a sensory impairment which limits the ability to feel pain or discomfort over 1/2 of body.
MOISTURE (degree to which skin is exposed to moisture)	**1. Constantly Moist:** Skin is kept moist almost constantly by perspiration, urine, etc. Dampness is detected every time patient is moved or turned.	**2. Very Moist:** Skin is often, but not always moist. Linen must be changed at least once a shift.
ACTIVITY (ability to change and control body position)	**1. Bedfast:** Confined to bed.	**2. Chairfast:** Ability to walk severely limited or non-existent. Cannot bear own weight and/or must be assisted into chair or wheelchair.
MOBILITY (ability to change and control body position)	**1. Completely Immobile:** Does not make even slight changes in body or extremity position without assistance.	**2. Very Limited:** Makes occasional slight changes in body or extremity position but unable to make frequent or significant changes independently.
NUTRITION (*usual* food intake value)	**1. Very poor:** Never eats a complete meal. Rarely eats more than 1/3 of any food offered. Eats 2 servings or less of protein (meat or dairy products) per day. Takes fluids poorly. Does not take liquid dietary supplement. **or** is NPO and/or maintained on clear liquids or IV's for more than 5 days.	**2. Probably Inadequate:** Rarely eats a complete meal and generally eats only about 1/2 of any food offered. Protein intake includes only 3 servings of meat or dairy products per day. Occasionally will take a dietary supplement. **or** receives less than optimum amount of liquid diet or tube feeding.
FRICTION AND SHEAR	**1. Problem:** Requires moderate to maximum assistance in moving. Complete lifting without sliding against sheets is impossible. Frequently slides down in bed or chair, requiring frequent repositioning with maximum assistance. Spasticity, contractures or agitation leads to almost constant friction.	**2. Potential Problem:** Moves feebly or requires minimum assistance. During a move skin probably slides to some extent against sheets, chair, restraints, or other devices. Maintains relatively good position in chair or bed most of the time but occasionally slides down.

Fig. 6-3
Braden Scale for predicting pressure sore risk. (Copyright © 1988 by Barbara Braden and Nancy Bergstrom. Used with permission.)

	Date of Assessment				

3. Slightly Limited:
Responds to verbal commands, but cannot always communicate discomfort or need to be turned.

or

has some impairment which limits ability to feel pain or discomfort in 1 or 2 extremities.

4. No Impairment:
Responds to verbal commands. Has no sensory deficit which would limit ability to feel or voice pain or discomfort.

3. Occasionally Moist:
Skin is occasionally moist, requiring an extra linen change approximately once a day.

4. Rarely Moist:
Skin is usually dry, linen only requires changing at routine intervals.

3. Walks Occasionally:
Walks occasionally during day, but for very short distances, with or without assistance. Spends majority of each shift in bed or chair.

4. Walks Frequently:
Walks outside the room at least twice a day and inside room at least once every 2 hours during waking hours.

3. Slightly Limited:
Makes frequent though slight changes in body or extremity position independently.

4. No Limitations:
Makes major and frequent changes in position without assistance.

3. Adequate:
Eats over half of most meals. Eats a total of 4 servings of protein (meat, dairy products) each day. Occasionally will refuse a meal, but will usually take a supplement if offered.

or

is on a tube feeding or TPN regimen which probably meets most of nutritional needs.

4. Excellent:
Eats most of every meal. Never refuses a meal. Usually eats a total of 4 or more servings of meat and dairy products. Occasionally eats between meals. Does not require supplementation.

3. No Apparent Problem:
Moves in bed and in chair independently and has sufficient muscle strength to lift up completely during move. Maintains good position in bed or chair at all times.

Total Score

Fig. 6-3, cont'd
Braden Scale for predicting pressure sore risk.

conceptual schema developed by Braden and Bergstrom (1987) identifies the intensity and duration of pressure and the tolerance of the skin and supporting structures to pressure as the critical determinants of pressure ulcers. Fig. 6-2 depicts those factors most often linked to pressure ulcer development.

Determining the older client's risk of pressure ulcer development should be part of skin assessment. The Braden scale (Fig. 6-3) for predicting pressure ulcer risk includes six subscales: sensory perception, moisture, activity, mobility, nutrition, and friction and shear. Each of the subscales rates factors within the above schema from 1 (least favorable) to 4 (most favorable), for a total of 23 points. A score of 16 points or less is the critical cutoff point for predicting risk.

Hair, nails, and glands constitute the epidermal appendages. Hair develops in one of the epidermal layers but eventually is embedded in the dermis. Each hair consists of a root, shaft, and follicle. Melanocytes in the shaft provide the color.

The quantity, quality, and distribution of hair change with age. There is a generalized loss of hair from the periphery to the center of the body. Hair of the scalp, extremities, axillae, and pubis decreases and thins. Pubic hair becomes less kinky and more gray. Hair in the nasal orifice, ear, and eyebrows becomes coarse and thick. There is a decrease in facial hair in men and an increase in women.

Nails are also formed in an epidermal layer. Nails protect the digits and, in the case of fingernails, aid in grasping small objects. Each nail consists of a body, free edge, and root. With age, nails grow more slowly and become thicker, tougher, more brittle, and less lustrous.

Glands originate in the epidermal layer but are located in the dermis, where they are physically and nutritionally supported. The glands of the skin are sebaceous, or oil glands, and eccrine and apocrine, or sweat glands.

Sebaceous glands are connected to a hair follicle because they develop from the follicular epithelium of the hair. These glands secrete sebum, which consists mostly of lipids, along the shaft of hair to the skin surface. Sebum lubricates and waterproofs the skin and keeps the hair from splitting and becoming brittle. The secretion of sebum is stimulated primarily by testosterone, so sebaceous gland activity decreases in both males and females as a result of the diminished hormonal levels that accompany advancing age.

Eccrine glands are found throughout the body, but they are more concentrated on the forehead, back, palms, and soles. These glands function in evaporative cooling in response to thermal or psychologic stimuli. The decreased number and activity of sweat glands with age cause an overall reduction of spontaneous sweating.

Apocrine glands are found only in the axillary and pubic regions, nipples and areolae, eyelids, and external ear. These glands are not functional until puberty. The characteristic adult body odor results from the products of bacterial decomposition of apocrine sweat. There are no apocrine gland changes associated with age.

Assessment of the Integument

Equipment needed:
    Transparent pocket ruler
    Penlight

Step	Normal/Individual Variations/Deviations
Skin	
Inspect color	Deep to light brown, whitish-pink to ruddy, olive or yellow overtones; sun-exposed areas, knees, and elbows may appear darker; senile lentigines on dorsal surface of hands, forearms, or face
	Hypopigmented patches; calloused areas may appear yellow
	DEVIATIONS: Marked yellowing, cyanosis, or erythema
Inspect and palpate moisture	Decreased perspiration
	Increased dryness, particularly extremities
	DEVIATIONS: Marked flaking
Palpate texture	Roughness on exposed areas or areas of pressure (elbows, knees, palms, soles)
	Flaking and scaling of dry skin areas

Continued

Step	Normal/Individual Variations/Deviations
Skin—cont'd	
	DEVIATIONS: Extensive or widespread roughness; excoriation over flaking, scaling areas; excessive thickening or hardening
Palpate temperature	Wide range of cool to warm
	DEVIATIONS: Excessively cold or warm, either generalized or localized
Inspect and palpate turgor	Overall increase in wrinkling, skinfolds, and laxness
	Sagging and drooping of pendulous parts
	DEVIATIONS: Excessive sagging of skinfolds and protruding of bony prominences (marked weight loss); excoriation of intertriginous areas
Note hygiene	Clean and odor-free
	Difficult-to-reach areas may be less clean
	DEVIATIONS: Crusted skin, foul body odor
Inspect, palpate, and measure lesions	See Table 6-3 for complete description
	DEVIATIONS: See Table 6-5 for complete description
Inspect, palpate, and measure trauma-induced lesions	Evidence of delayed healing of bruises, lacerations, and excoriation
	DEVIATIONS: Skin tears, particularly on extremities; excessive bruises, lacerations, or excoriation
Inspect and palpate bony prominences of partially or totally immobilized client (Fig. 6-4)	Redness returns to original skin color when pressure relieved; skin intact
	Pressure point temperature equal to surrounding skin temperature
	DEVIATIONS: Hyperemia extends over a long period; stage I to IV pressure sore (Table 6-6); pressure point warmer than surrounding skin

Continued on p. 115

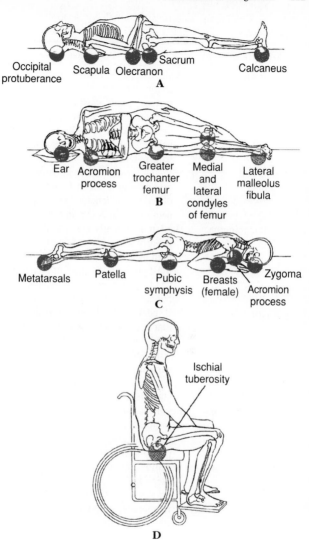

Fig. 6-4
Bony prominences vulnerable to pressure. **A,** Supine. **B,** Side-lying. **C,** Prone. **D,** Sitting. (Modified from Forbes EJ, Fitzsimons VM: *The older adult: a process for wellness,* St Louis, 1981, Mosby.)

Table 6-5   Commonly occurring abnormal skin lesions in older people

Skin Lesion	Description
Actinic or senile keratosis	Whitish to erythematous macular lesion with irregular, rough, scaly surface; found most commonly on the dorsal surfaces of the hands, arms, neck, face, scalp, pinnae, and any sun-exposed areas; has malignant potential
Squamous cell carcinoma	Soft, red-brown nodule in early stage; progressing to ulcer; found most often on lips, cheek, ear, temple, or neck, but can occur anywhere
Basal cell carcinoma	Hard, red, or pearly gray papular lesion in early stage, progressing to ulcer with bleeding and crusting; found most often on "T-zone" of face (forehead, eyelids, cheeks, nose, and lips), but can occur anywhere
Herpes zoster	Red, edematous plaques or vesicles that become filled with purulent fluid; vesicles eventually weep and crust; occur most commonly along a dermatome of thorax, abdomen, forehead and temple, neck, and shoulders
Seborrheic dermatitis	Erythematous rash commonly found on forehead, face, and upper chest that may erupt into red-brown papules with yellowish scaling
Malignant melanoma	Variation in color (red, white, and blue areas within a brown-black lesion) on any area of skin or mucous membrane; irregular border and irregular surface topography

Table 6-5   Commonly occurring abnormal skin lesions
in older people—cont'd

Skin Lesion	Description
Candidiasis	Shiny, red, macerated plaques outlined by pustules and papules with satellite lesions; found in warm, moist, intertriginous skin areas; etiology is *Candida albicans* fungus
Scabies	Fine, wavy, dark lines under the skin, occurring predominantly between the fingers, but also on inner surfaces of thighs and forearms, about the elbows and axillary folds, under breasts, and around the perineum; secondary bacterial infection may occur; etiology is *Sarcoptes scabiei,* the itch mite
Pediculosis capitis (head lice)	Small, ovoid, grayish white nits (ova) are fixed to the hair shaft, sometimes in great numbers; may be found around the occiput and behind the ears; sometimes involve the eyebrows, eyelashes, and beard; severe itching can cause excoriation of scalp with secondary bacterial infection
Pediculosis corporis (body lice)	Wheal with central hemorrhagic spot caused by bites, usually associated with linear scratch marks, urticaria, or superficial bacterial infection; later presentation is dry, scaly pigmentation

Table 6-6   Criteria for staging pressure sores

Skin is intact: no apparent skin problems, no area of redness.

Stage I	Nonblanchable erythema of intact skin; the heralding lesion of skin ulceration. NOTE: Reactive hyperemia can normally be expected to be present for one-half to three-fourths as long as the pressure occluded blood flow to the area; it should not be confused with a stage I pressure ulcer.
Stage II	Partial thickness skin loss involving epidermis and/or dermis. The ulcer is superficial and presents clinically as an abrasion, blister, or shallow crater.
Stage III	Full-thickness skin loss involving damage or necrosis of subcutaneous tissue that may extend down to, but not through, underlying fascia. The ulcer presents clinically as a deep crater with or without undermining of adjacent tissue.
Stage IV	Full-thickness skin loss with extensive destruction, tissue necrosis, or damage to muscle, bone, or supporting structures (for example, tendon or joint capsule). NOTE: Undermining and sinus tracts may also be associated with stage IV pressure ulcers.

Staging definitions recognize these limitations:
- Assessment of stage I pressure ulcers may be difficult in patients with darkly pigmented skin.
- When eschar is present, accurate staging of the pressure ulcer is not possible until the eschar has sloughed or the wound has been debrided.

From Panel on the Prediction and Prevention of Pressure Ulcers in Adults: Pressure ulcers in adults: prediction and prevention. In *Quick reference guide for clinicians,* AHCPR Publication No. 92-0050, Rockville, Md, 1992, Agency for Health Care Policy and Research, Public Health Service, US Department of Health and Human Services.

Step	Normal/Individual Variations/Deviations

Hair

Inspect color

Wide variations from white to gray hair on scalp, body, pubic area, axillae, and face

True color may be altered with rinses or dyes

Inspect quantity and distribution

Scalp, body, pubic, axillary, and facial hair sparse and thin (facial hair increased in women)

Symmetric balding in men

DEVIATIONS: Sudden hair loss; patchy balding

Inspect and palpate texture

Dry, brittle scalp hair

Coarse facial, nasal orifice, and ear hair and eyebrows

Fine body hair

Less kinky pubic hair

DEVIATIONS: Excessive dryness and brittleness of scalp hair

Nails

Inspect color of toenails and fingernails

Variations of pink; dark-skinned persons may have pigment deposits; yellowish color

Diminished transparency

DEVIATIONS: Cyanotic, excessively yellow, splinter hemorrhages

Inspect and palpate shape

Some distortion of normal flat or slightly curved surface

DEVIATIONS: Spoon shape (associated with hypochromic anemias, chronic infections, malnutrition, Raynaud's disease); clubbing

Inspect and palpate consistency

Thick, brittle, peeling

DEVIATIONS: Excessive thickening (associated with psoriasis, fungal infection, defective vascular supply)

Sample Documentation—Herpes Zoster

Health History

Mrs. G., 78, reports 3-day duration of slight tingling sensation across right shoulder blade, around to area just below right breast; associated with mild redness and a burning sensation; adds she doesn't feel her usual energetic self. Woke up this morning and noted a rash over this same area, with a few clusters of tiny blisters and "severe" pain. Can't tolerate anything touching the affected area. Only medications include daily multivitamin and a calcium supplement.

Physical Examination

Unilateral band of bright red erythema at about T4-T5 level, with a maculopapular rash and several small clusters of 2 to 4 mm fluid-filled vesicles; no rupturing of vesicles noted. No lymphadenopathy. Area is extremely tender to light touch.

Client Teaching

Prevention and Treatment of Dry Skin (Xerosis)

1. Restrict use of harsh soap for bathing, particularly deodorant soap. Be sure to rinse thoroughly to remove excess soap.
2. Bathe 2 to 3 times a week using *tepid* water rather than hot water.
3. Apply an unscented lanolin-containing emollient after bathing (while skin is still moist) to help retain moisture absorbed while bathing. Expensive products are not necessarily better than cheaper ones.

Compiled from *Skin Care and Aging:* Age page, National Institute on Aging, Bethesda, Md, 1991, US Department of Health and Human Services, Public Health Service, National Institutes of Health.

Client Teaching—cont'd

4. Use room humidifiers or place pans of water over heating elements to increase moisture in environment. Keep room temperature at a comfortable level without making it too hot.
5. Avoid bath oil because of the risk of slipping in the tub. Oil may be added to rinse water for undergarments and bed linens if desired.
6. Avoid wearing rough fabrics next to skin; wear cotton undergarments.
7. If self-treatment for dryness and itching is not effective, consult health care practitioner; skin condition may be a symptom of underlying disease.

References

Braden B, Bergstrom B: A conceptual schema for the study of the etiology of pressure sores, *Rehab Nurs* 12(1):9,1987.

Forbes EJ, Fitzsimons VM: *The older adult: a process for wellness,* St Louis, 1981, Mosby.

Gilchrest BA: Skin diseases in the elderly. In Calkins E et al, eds: *The practice of geriatrics,* Philadelphia, 1986, Saunders.

Potter PA: *Pocket guide to health assessment,* ed 3, St Louis, 1994, Mosby.

Skin Care and Aging: Age page, National Institute on Aging, Bethesda, Md, 1991, US Department of Health and Human Services, Public Health Service, National Institutes of Health.

Thompson JM: *Clinical outlines for health assessment,* St Louis, 1997, Mosby.

Assessment of the Head, Face, and Neck

7

Although there are many structures located in the head and neck area to study, this chapter focuses only on the structural components of the head (skull and face) and neck (thyroid gland, trachea, and lymphatic nodes). Portions of assessment of other head and neck structures presented in other chapters are integrated with the head and neck regions when the complete physical examination is conducted.

The skills of inspection, palpation, and auscultation are used in assessing the head, face, and neck. Equipment needs include a stethoscope, transparent pocket ruler, and cup of water.

Anatomy and Physiology

Head and Face

The skull, consisting of cranial and facial bones, contains several cavities that house the brain and sensory organs. Variations in bone shape and density result in wide differences in individual skull size and facial appearance. The cranium includes one frontal, two parietal, two temporal, and one occipital bone, all covered by the scalp with variable amounts of hair. Regions of the head are named from these underlying structures (Fig. 7-1).

The head contains the salivary glands that produce and secrete saliva. Saliva contains enzymes that digest starch and fat, as well as mucus that lubricates the oral cavity to facilitate swallowing. Saliva also cleanses the teeth. The three major pairs of salivary glands are the parotid, submandibular, and sublingual.

Overall salivary gland activity decreases with advanced age, resulting in dryness of the mouth and reduced ability to protect the

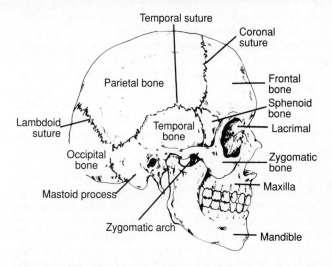

Fig. 7-1
Anatomic landmarks of the skull. (From Thompson JM: *Clinical outlines for health assessment,* St Louis, 1997, Mosby.)

gums from irritation. An increase in the mucin component of salivary mucus causes saliva to thicken and become ropy in texture, diminishing the natural cleansing action of saliva.

The facial bones include the mandible and two nasal, two maxilla, two lacrimal, and two zygomatic bones (Fig. 7-1). The mandible is attached to the skull by a temporomandibular articulation and is the only movable facial bone. The remaining fused facial bones form the basic shape of the face, support the teeth, and provide attachments for various muscles that move the jaw and enable the formation of facial expressions.

The palpebral fissures and nasolabial folds are the major facial landmarks. The normal facies of the older adult is affected by nutritional status, by systemic and local conditions, and by the degree of awareness and interest. Wrinkles are more prominent at the corners of the eyes. Resorption of orbital fat and laxness of surrounding tissue result in ptosis or drooping of the lids and suborbital puffiness. Nasolabial folds become more prominent, extend toward the chin, and create jowls. However, an edentulous state is associated with mandibular resorption, shrinkage of the lower portion of the face, and infolding of the mouth.

Facial muscles are innervated by cranial nerves V (trigeminal) and VII (facial). The function of these nerves is also tested as part of the neurologic examination (see Chapter 17) but is usually carried out at this time.

The major accessible artery of the face is the temporal artery, which passes just anterior to the ear over the temporal muscle and onto the forehead. It is palpable just anterior to the tragus of the ear.

Neck

The physical structure of the neck is formed by the cervical vertebrae and the trapezius and sternocleidomastoid muscles. The relationship of these muscles to each other and to adjacent bones creates the anterior and posterior triangles of the neck that are used as anatomic landmarks (Fig. 7-2). The anterior triangle is between the right and left sternocleidomastoid muscles, with the mandible forming the superior boundary. The trachea, thyroid gland, and anterior cervical lymph nodes lie within this triangle. The carotid artery lies anterior and parallel to the sternocleidomastoid muscle. The posterior triangle lies between the sternocleidomastoid and

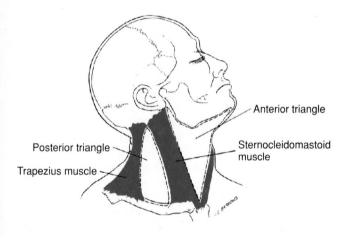

Anterior triangle

Sternocleidomastoid muscle

Posterior triangle

Trapezius muscle

Fig. 7-2
The trapezius and sternocleidomastoid muscles and the anterior and posterior triangles. (From Malasanos L et al: *Health assessment,* ed 4, St Louis, 1990, Mosby.)

trapezius muscles. The posterior cervical lymph nodes are found here. The size, symmetry, and strength of the trapezius and sterno-cleidomastoid muscles are evaluated by testing cranial nerve XI (spinal accessory).

Height loss associated with age occurs primarily as a result of changes in the vertebral column. These make the neck curve backward, which shortens the distance between the occiput and shoulder. An accumulation of fat around the cervical vertebrae, particularly in women, creates a "dowager's hump."

Two prominent wrinkle lines appear on either side of the midline of the neck. Sagging of surrounding tissue and deposition of fat give the appearance of a double chin.

The trachea connects the larynx to the bronchus and is located in the central anterior neck. C-shaped rings of hyaline cartilage form the walls of the trachea, with the open part of the C lying posteriorly. The cricoid cartilage ring connects the thyroid cartilage above and the trachea below (Fig. 7-3). No normal age-related changes occur in the trachea.

The thyroid gland lies in the lower anterior neck below the thyroid cartilage. This gland consists of a right lobe and a left lobe

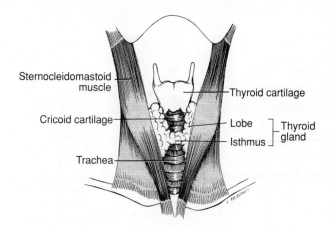

Fig. 7-3

The thyroid gland lies anteriorly in the neck. It is fixed to the sides of the trachea, and its isthmus overlies the trachea. (From Potter PA: *Pocket guide to health assessment,* ed 3, St Louis, 1994, Mosby.)

that lie on either side of the trachea and that are connected by an isthmus. The extreme lateral portions are covered by the sterno-cleidomastoid muscles (Fig. 7-3). The thyroid is an endocrine gland that regulates metabolism in all organs. Thyroxine (T_4), tri-iodothyronine (T_3), and calcitonin are the major hormones se-creted by the thyroid. T_4 and T_3 control metabolic rate, regulate growth, and stimulate nervous and cardiac activity. Calcitonin regulates serum calcium levels.

As a result of age-related changes in stature, including changes in the neck, the thyroid gland may move to a lower position in re-lation to the clavicles. The gland itself becomes more flexible, which may increase its nodularity on palpation.

Lymph nodes are small, round, or oval bodies usually found in clusters in specific regions of the body. In the head and neck, there are numerous lymph nodes filtering lymphatic fluid from these ar-eas (Fig. 7-4). The lymph nodes contain B and T lymphocytes, which are responsible for immunity, and phagocytes, which filter foreign particles and cellular debris from lymph. The size of

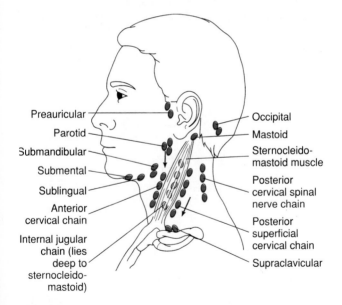

Fig. 7-4
Lymph nodes of the head and neck. (From Barkauskas VH et al: *Health and physical assessment,* ed 2, St Louis, 1998, Mosby.)

lymph nodes decreases with advanced age because of loss of some of the lymphoid elements. Nodes also become fibrotic and fatty, which is thought to possibly diminish the older person's ability to resist infection.

Assessment of the Head, Face, and Neck

NOTE: Ask client to remove wigs, hair pieces, or toupees.
Equipment needed:
    Stethoscope
    Transparent pocket ruler
    Cup of water

Step	Normal/Individual Variations/Deviations
Inspect and palpate:	
Skull for size, shape, contour, and position	Size proportional to overall body size
	Ovoid shape with long diameter on anteroposterior axis; symmetric and smooth with prominent frontal, occipital areas
	Head may be tilted backward slightly
	DEVIATIONS: Marked enlargement overall in relation to facial bones, increased length of mandible; lateral expansion of skull; gross asymmetry; swelling or depressions
Scalp for color, texture, lesions, hygiene, tenderness (NOTE: Part hair in several areas; assess lesions in same manner as for skin lesions.)	Color consistent with other, unexposed areas
	Smooth texture
	Clean without lesions or infections
	Nontender
	DEVIATIONS: Uneven pigmentation; lesions, excessive scaliness or dryness; nits, lice; tenderness

Continued

Step	Normal/Individual Variations/Deviations
Face for color, proportions, expression, movements	Even color distribution Spacing and symmetry consistent with genetic heritage; minor asymmetries Alert and interested with smooth, expressive movements Smooth movements that correspond to conversation DEVIATIONS: Increased pigmentation, jaundice, cyanosis, extreme paleness; striking enlargements of facial bones, marked asymmetry; dull, sleepy, masklike, tense, overexcited; tics, tremors, or twitches
Assess trigeminal (CN V) motor function **Technique:** Instruct client to clench teeth while examiner palpates muscles over jaw.	Bilaterally equal muscle contractions DEVIATIONS: Unequal muscle contractions; pain, fasciculations
Assess facial (CN VII) motor function **Technique:** Instruct client to raise eyebrows, close eyes tightly, frown, smile, show teeth, and puff out cheeks.	Symmetric facial movements DEVIATIONS: Gross asymmetry; tics; unilateral mouth drooping; flattening of nasolabial fold; laxity of lower eyelid
Palpate temporal artery	Regular rhythm, slightly diminished amplitude; soft, pliable, and nontender DEVIATIONS: Tender, tortuous, enlarged

Step	Normal/Individual Variations/Deviations
Assess spinal accessory (CN XI) function **Technique:** Instruct client to shrug shoulders against resistance of examiner's hands.	Strong, symmetric contraction of trapezius muscles DEVIATIONS: Gross unilateral or bilateral muscle weakness; pain or discomfort
Instruct client to turn head to one side against the resistance of examiner's hand.	Contraction of opposite sternocleidomastoid muscle; bilaterally equal force of movement against hand DEVIATIONS: Unable to oppose resistance of hand; asymmetric movement
Inspect neck for symmetry, movement and curvature, range of motion (NOTE: When evaluating range of motion, proceed slowly and judge each movement separately.)	Bilateral symmetry of sternocleidomastoid and trapezius muscles; nonwebbed appearance Smooth and coordinated movements Dorsal kyphosis and associated backward tilt of neck Women may exhibit dowager's hump because of accumulation of fat around cervical vertebrae DEVIATIONS: Asymmetry or unusual shortness; tics, spasms; decreased or absent cervical concavity
Technique (Range of motion): 1. Flex neck with chin toward sternum.	Reduced flexion ($<70°$)
2. Extend neck with chin pointing toward ceiling.	Reduced extension ($<30°$)

Continued

Step	Normal/Individual Variations/Deviations
3. Bend neck laterally with ear toward shoulder (right and left).	Reduced lateral bending (<35° from midline)
4. Rotate neck with chin toward shoulder (right and left).	Reduced rotation (<70° from midline) DEVIATIONS: Marked limitation of movement or pain with these maneuvers
Inspect and palpate trachea for location **Technique:** Place index and middle fingers along each side of trachea at suprasternal notch and note space between it and the sternocleidomastoid.	Midline at the suprasternal notch DEVIATIONS: Deviation from midline
Inspect thyroid for masses and symmetry (Ask client to take sip of water and swallow with neck slightly extended; observe movement of gland.)	Usually not visible on swallowing DEVIATIONS: Unilateral or bilateral lobe enlargement
Palpate thyroid for size, shape, consistency, nodules (NOTE: Locate landmarks [thyroid cartilage, cricoid cartilage, and tracheal rings] before palpating [Fig. 7-3].)	

Step	Normal/Individual Variations/Deviations
Technique (posterior approach):	
1. With client's head slightly extended, place fingertips of both hands just below cricoid cartilage. As client sips water and swallows, attempt to palpate the isthmus and lateral lobes.	Isthmus either not palpable or has smooth consistency Lobes either not palpable, or smooth borders freely rise with swallowing
2. Slightly turn client's head toward side to be examined, with chin slightly lowered. To examine right lobe, push with fingers of left hand to displace thyroid cartilage toward the right. Place right thumb behind sterno-cleidomastoid and palpating fingers in front. As client sips water and swallows, palpate right lobe as it slides between fingers and thumbs. Use same procedure to examine left side, but reverse position of hands (Fig. 7-5).	May feel slightly nodular or irregular because of fibrosis secondary to advanced age Nontender **DEVIATIONS:** Enlarged lobes; easily palpable without swallowing; tender

Continued

Step	Normal/Individual Variations/Deviations
Inspect and palpate lymph nodes: preauricular, postauricular (mastoid), occipital, parotid, sub-mandibular, sublingual, submental, anterior cervical, posterior cervical, deep cervical chain, supraclavicular	

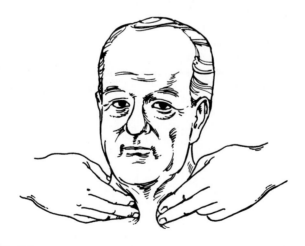

Fig. 7-5
Posterior approach for palpation of the thyroid gland. (Courtesy Karen L. Merrill.)

Step	Normal/Individual Variations/Deviations
Note size and shape, consistency, delimitation, fixation to surrounding tissues, tenderness, inflammation **Technique:** Using finger pads of index and middle fingers, move skin over underlying nodes while client's neck is slightly flexed toward side to be examined; compare one side to the other.	Not palpable DEVIATIONS: Palpable; large, firm, hard, nodular, irregular; discrete or matted together; fixed to underlying or overlying tissue; direct or referred tenderness; increased erythema, heat

Sample Documentation—Sialadenitis

Health History

Mr. L, 68, reports sudden onset of left-sided, nonradiating facial pain associated with cheek swelling. Took two extra-strength acetaminophen tablets four times yesterday and noted only mild relief of pain. Denies erythema or heat over affected area; no injury or trauma. Pain not affected by ingestion of hot, cold, or sweet substances. Denies dry eyes or dry mouth. Temperature 100° F.

Physical Examination

Mild degree of left-sided facial swelling; upper posterior maxillary area tender to light external palpation. Teeth and gingiva in good repair. No discharge noted from Stensen's duct on palpation of left parotid gland, but gland is tender and swollen; approximately 3 mm hard lump palpated in duct. No additional lymphadenopathy.

References

Barkauskas VH et al: *Health and physical assessment,* ed 3, St Louis, 1998, Mosby.

Malasanos L et al: *Health assessment,* ed 4, St Louis, 1990, Mosby.

Potter PA: *Pocket guide to health assessment,* ed 3, St Louis, 1994, Mosby.

Thompson JM: *Clinical outlines for health assessment,* St Louis, 1997, Mosby.

Assessment of the Eyes

8

Assessment of the eyes readily reveals to the examiner many clues to the physical and emotional status of the client. Because of the complexity and multiple components of the eye examination, the nurse must approach eye assessment systematically. An effective method is to begin with testing visual acuity and visual fields, then proceed to assessment of extraocular muscle (EOM) function, followed by assessment of external and internal structures. The assessment is completed with ophthalmoscopic examination. Inspection is the principal skill used in eye assessment. Equipment needs include a Snellen or "E" chart, Rosenbaum chart, opaque card, penlight, cotton wisp, cotton-tipped applicator, and ophthalmoscope.

Anatomy and Physiology

The eyes are the sensory organs that transmit stimuli through pathways in the brain to the occipital lobes, where the sense of vision is perceived. The ocular orbit, comprising portions of the facial bones, is cushioned with fat and is the bony framework that supports and protects the eyeball. This orbital fat resorbs with aging, leading to ptosis and enophthalmos. The accessory structures of eyelids, eyelashes, eyebrows, conjunctivae, lacrimal apparatus, and extraocular muscles provide additional protection (Figs. 8-1 and 8-2).

External Eye

The eyelids are folds of skin with attached muscle that allows them to move. The eyelids protect the eyeballs by reflexively blinking and moving lubricating fluid over the surface of the eyes. When the eyes are open and the client is gazing straight ahead, the

131

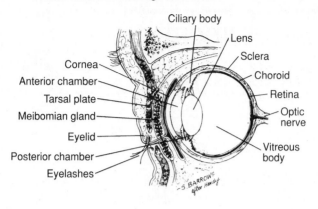

Fig. 8-1
Structures of the eyelid and globe. (From Malasanos L et al: *Health assessment,* ed 4, St Louis, 1990, Mosby.)

upper eyelid covers a small portion of the iris, and the lower lid meets the iris. The palpebral fissure is the opening between the upper and lower eyelids. Eyelashes on the edges of the lids prevent airborne objects from entering the eyes. Entropion, in which the eyelid turns inward so the lashes rub against the eye, causes corneal abrasion. Ectropion, in which the eyelid turns outward, prevents normal closure and causes redness and congestion of the eyeball. Both of these abnormal positions may result from tissue laxity secondary to aging or to scarring of the eyelids as a result of infection.

Eyebrows are located transversely above both eyes along the superior orbital ridges of the skull. These short, thick hairs prevent perspiration from entering the eyes. With age, the brows may turn gray, may become coarser in men, and may thin at the temporal sides in both men and women.

The conjunctiva, a thin, transparent mucus-secreting membrane, is divided into two portions: the palpebral conjunctiva, which lines the interior surface of each eyelid and appears shiny pink or red, and the bulbar conjunctiva, which lines the anterior surface of the eyeball up to the limbus and appears clear. With age, the conjunctiva thins and takes on a yellowish appearance. Pingueculae, small, yellow, fatty nodules on the bulbar conjunctiva near the limbus, are often seen.

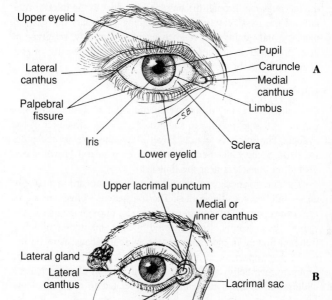

Fig. 8-2

A, Anterior view of the eye. **B,** Lacrimal system. (**A** from Barkauskas, VH et al: *Health and physical assessment,* ed 2, St. Louis, 1998, Mosby; **B** From Thompson JM et al: *Mosby's manual of clinical nursing,* ed 3, St Louis, 1993, Mosby.)

The lacrimal apparatus consists of the lacrimal glands, ducts, and puncta (Fig. 8-2, *B*). The lacrimal gland is located in the superolateral portion of the orbit and is innervated by cranial nerve VII (facial). The gland produces tears, which moisten and lubricate the conjunctiva and cornea. As the eyelid blinks, tears pass over the eye and drain into the puncta. The tears drain from the puncta into the lacrimal sac through the nasolacrimal duct to the inferior meatus of the nasal cavity. With advancing age, tears decrease in quantity and quality and tend to evaporate quickly, resulting in drier conjunctivae. Excessive tearing may occur because of impaired drainage of the ductal system.

Internal Eye

The sclera or "white" of the eye is composed of elastic and collagen fibers that give shape to and protect the inner structures of the eyeball. The sclera is avascular, yet it contains sensory receptors for pain. Some older persons may develop scleral brown spots, visible on the sclera near the limbus.

The anterior portion of the sclera extends outward in a convex curve and becomes the cornea. The transparent, convex nature of the cornea permits the transmission of light through the lens to the retina. The cornea is often yellowed by age, and arcus senilis is a frequent finding in older persons. Arcus senilis consists of fat deposits that appear as an arc or circle a few millimeters from the limbus. Once believed to be associated with an elevated plasma cholesterol level, arcus senilis is not related to any pathologic disorder.

The lens separates the eyeball into two cavities: the anterior and posterior chambers. The anterior chamber is located in front of the iris and behind the cornea. The posterior chamber is located between the iris and the lens. Both chambers connect through the pupil and are filled with aqueous humor, which is produced by the ciliary body. Regulation of aqueous production and outflow determines intraocular pressure. Glaucoma, an eye disease frequently associated with aging, refers to an increased intraocular pressure.

The iris is a pigmented, round disk surrounded by smooth muscle fibers. The contraction of these muscle fibers regulates the diameter of the pupil, an opening in the center of the iris. With age, the pupil decreases in size and loses the ability to constrict in response to light and accommodation.

The lens is a transparent structure lying directly behind the iris. The lens is supported and its shape controlled by muscles of the ciliary body. Changes in thickness of the lens determine the amount of light reaching the retina and the focusing of objects on the retina. The lens yellows with age and gradually becomes more opaque, resulting in cataract formation.

The retina is the innermost layer of the eye where visual images are projected. Retinal structures visible with ophthalmoscopy include the optic disc, or nerve head of the optic nerve; the four sets of retinal vessels that emanate from the optic disc and travel medially and laterally around the retina; the macula, where central vision and color perception are concentrated; and the reddish orange retinal background itself (Fig. 8-3). The physiologic cup is the small depression within the disc itself, located just temporal to the center of the disc and occupying one fourth to one third of the total area of the disc.

The following are signs of aging that may be observed. Blood vessels become narrower and straighter. Arteries may appear more opaque and somewhat gray in color. Drusen, localized areas of hyaline degeneration, will appear as small, round, gray or yellow spots near the macula.

The external and internal age-related eye changes just noted may affect the older person's functional ability. Vision in dimly lit areas and adaptation to darkness are reduced, while glare can cause pain and limit the ability to clearly distinguish objects. Yellowing of the lens affects ability to accurately perceive and distinguish colors: soft pastels (blue, pink, green) appear the same and dark colors (navy blue, maroon, brown, black) appear the same. A decrease in peripheral vision and alterations in depth perception combine to place the older person at risk for injury.

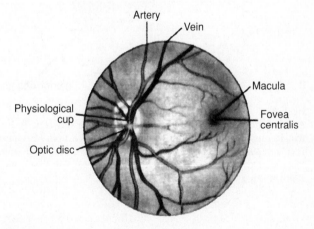

Fig. 8-3
Retinal landmarks. (From Thompson JM, Bowers AC: *Health assessment: an illustrated pocket guide,* ed 3, St Louis, 1992, Mosby.)

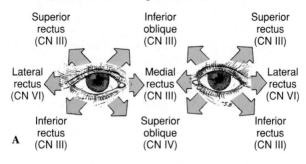

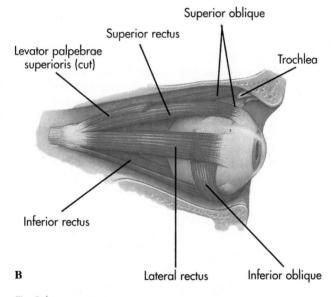

Fig. 8-4

A, Movement generated by the six extraocular muscles. **B,** Extrinsic muscles of the right eye, lateral view. (**A** from Malasanos L et al: *Health assessment,* ed 4, St Louis, 1990, Mosby; **B** from Thibodeau GA, Patton KT: *Anatomy & physiology,* ed 3, St Louis, 1996, Mosby.)

Extraocular Muscles

The movements of the eyeball are controlled by six extrinsic eye muscles: the superior, inferior, lateral, and medial rectus muscles and the superior and inferior oblique muscles (Fig. 8-4). The eyes move in the same direction because the muscle of one eye works with a corresponding muscle of the other eye. The six eye muscles are innervated by three cranial nerves. The oculomotor nerve (CN III) innervates the medial, superior, and inferior rectus muscles and the inferior oblique muscle. The trochlear nerve (CN IV) innervates the superior oblique muscle, and the abducens nerve (CN VI) innervates the lateral rectus muscle.

Assessment of the Eyes

Equipment needed:

Snellen chart	Cotton wisp
Rosenbaum chart	Cotton-tipped applicator
Opaque card	Ophthalmoscope
Penlight	

Step	Normal/Individual Variations/Deviations
Assess visual acuity (CN II): Measure distant vision **Technique:** Place Snellen chart 20 feet from client in an evenly bright, well-lit room. Test each eye individually, asking client to cover one eye with opaque card. Ask client to read the letters in the line the client sees best. Determine smallest line in which client identifies all the letters and record acuity at that line. Repeat with other eye. Test with and without glasses, but without glasses first.	20/20 to 20/30 OU with corrective lenses DEVIATION: Any line above the 20/30 line on the chart

Continued

Step	Normal/Individual Variations/Deviations
Measure near vision **Technique:** Ask client to hold Rosenbaum chart 14 inches from face at eye level. Test and record vision as with Snellen chart. Presbyopic clients should read through bifocal segment of glasses.	As described above DEVIATION: As described above
Assess visual fields by confrontation (CN II) **Technique:** Sit or stand opposite client at eye level, 1½ to 2 feet apart. Ask client to cover right eye with opaque card while examiner covers left eye. Stare straight at each other. Examiner fully extends arm midway between client and self, gradually progressing toward the midline with fingers moving. Instruct client to indicate when the moving fingers are first seen. Compare client's response to your own. Repeat to test superior, inferior, and temporal fields. Repeat entire procedure with other eye covered. (NOTE: This is a gross measurement that assumes the examiner has normal visual fields.)	Client and examiner see moving fingers at same time: Nasally: 60° Superiorly: 50° Inferiorly: 70° Temporally: 90° DEVIATION: Client does not see moving fingers at same time as examiner

Step	Normal/Individual Variations/Deviations
Assess extraocular muscle functions:	
Six cardinal fields of gaze (CN III, IV, VI)	Smooth, coordinated movements through all six positions; no divergence in any position
Technique: Ask client to hold head in a fixed position and have only eyes follow examiner's finger as it moves through the six cardinal fields (Fig. 8-4, *A*).	DEVIATIONS: Jerky, uncoordinated movement in any position; sustained nystagmus
Ask client to look at extreme temporal-lateral positions while examiner holds finger in those positions momentarily.	A few beats of end-positional nystagmus DEVIATION: Sustained nystagmus
Corneal light reflex	Light reflected symmetrically from both pupils
Technique: Ask client to stare straight ahead as examiner shines a penlight on nasal bridge from a distance of 12 to 15 inches.	DEVIATION: Asymmetric light reflections in each eye
Cover-uncover test	Uncovered eye does not move while card placed over other eye; newly uncovered eye does not move
Technique: Ask client to stare straight ahead at a near fixed point. Cover one of client's eyes with opaque card and observe uncovered eye for movement to focus on designated point. Remove cover and observe eye just uncovered for same movement. Repeat procedure with other eye.	DEVIATIONS: Movement of uncovered eye to focus on fixed point; newly uncovered eye moves to focus

Continued

Step	Normal/Individual Variations/Deviations
Assess ocular structures	
Inspect eyelids for position and color, closure, height of palpebral fissures, blinking, and position of globe	Symmetric position with varying degrees of upper lid drooping; color consistent with body skin, no redness
	Bilaterally equal palpebral fissure height
	Frequent involuntary movements bilaterally
	Symmetric placement of globe; slight enophthalmos
	DEVIATIONS: Excessive lid drooping interfering with vision; asymmetric position; rapid blinking, blepharospasm, staring; asymmetric placement; marked enophthalmos or exophthalmos
Inspect eyebrows for quantity, condition, and distribution of hair, and for movement	Moderate thinning, especially at temporal side; coarse
	Brows symmetrically shaped along bony prominence above orbit; symmetric lifting of brows
	DEVIATIONS: Scant density or complete absence; asymmetric brows
Inspect and palpate lacrimal gland, puncta, and ducts for edema, tenderness, redness, discharge (Fig. 8-2, *B*)	Pink, no erythema in area of puncta or ducts; without edema, redness, tenderness, exudate or fluid
	Gland nontender
	DEVIATIONS: Redness, edema, tenderness, discharge, excessive dryness, or tearing

Step	Normal/Individual Variations/Deviations
Inspect sclera and conjunctiva for color, vascular pattern, lesions, edema **Technique:** Separate lid widely with thumb and index finger exerting pressure against ridge of bony orbit surrounding eye; ask client to look up, down, and to each side. Repeat procedure with other eye. Inspect upper tarsal conjunctiva only if foreign body suspected. **Technique:** Ask client to look down with eye slightly open, while gently pulling upper eyelashes downward and forward, to break suction between lid and globe. Next, evert lid by placing a small cotton-tipped applicator about 1 cm above eyelid margin; gently push downward with applicator while still holding upper lashes. Inspect and remove any foreign body that may be present. Return eyelid to its normal position by having client look up and blink.	White sclera; brown spots near limbus Bulbar conjunctiva somewhat dry in appearance; clear with small vessels visible; pingueculae may be present near limbus Palpebral conjunctiva light pink without lesions or discharge DEVIATIONS: Excessively yellow or dark blue; increased number and size of visible vessels; pale or excessively red; lesions, discharge; foreign body

Continued

Step	Normal/Individual Variations/Deviations
Inspect cornea for transparency and surface characteristics **Technique:** Direct penlight obliquely from several positions.	Transparent, smoothly rounded, clear; often yellow; arcus senilis may be present Symmetric blink reflex DEVIATIONS: Cloudy or opaque; pigmentation; abrasions or ulcerations on surface; pterygium; failure of blink reflex unilaterally or bilaterally
Test corneal sensitivity (CN V) **Technique:** Instruct client to keep eyes open and look up and away while you lightly touch cornea with a fine cotton wisp.	
Inspect anterior chamber, using oblique lighting technique described above, for transparency and iris surface and depth	Transparent Iris flat Slightly shallow but with clearance between cornea and iris maintained DEVIATIONS: Any visible material; bulging forward, evident by shadow cast on iris; marked shallowness
Inspect iris for color and shape	Symmetric, but may be somewhat dull Round, smooth, slightly concave Wedge or portion may be missing secondary to cataract removal DEVIATIONS: Inconsistency between eyes; irregular shape

Step	Normal/Individual Variations/Deviations
Inspect pupil for size and shape	Round, symmetric, neither widely dilated nor pinpoint under normal lighting conditions; overall slightly smaller with advanced age
Test reaction to light and accommodation (CN III) **Technique:** Have room dimly lit. Instruct client to keep both eyes open and look straight ahead while you approach with penlight from one side and shine light directly on pupil. Repeat procedure with other eye.	Prompt constriction of illuminated pupil (direct response) and simultaneous constriction of other pupil (consensual response) DEVIATIONS: Unequal size (anisocoria); irregular shape; absent or unequal response
Instruct client to look at a distant object. Hold up object (finger, penlight) approximately 10 cm from bridge of client's nose. Ask client to focus eyes on the near object.	Pupils converge and symmetrically constrict as eyes focus on near object DEVIATION: Absent or unequal convergence or constriction
Assess retinal structures with the ophthalmoscope (see the box on p. 146) Red reflex	Red or red-orange glow in pupil; glow may be interrupted by dark spots or black shadows indicating opacities DEVIATION: Decrease in or absence of red reflex resulting from cataract or hemorrhage into vitreous humor

Continued

Step	Normal/Individual Variations/Deviations
Optic disc for size, shape, color, cup, and margins	Approximately 1.5 mm in diameter
	Round, oval
	Pale reddish yellow to creamy pink; color darker in dark-skinned people
	Smooth, gray central area of disc
	Temporal margin sharp, nasal margin less defined; gray or dark crescent on temporal margin
	DEVIATIONS: Blurred margins; bilaterally unequal size and shape; diffuse pallor; excessively pale; occupying more than half of the disc's diameter
Retinal vessels	Arterioles smaller in diameter (ratio 2:3 or 4:5) than accompanying venules
	Narrow light streak in center of arteriole; arterioles may appear more opaque, gray in color, and narrower
	Venules darker in color (purplish red) with patchy or no light reflection
	Arteriolar-venule crossings should not alter caliber of underlying vessel
	DEVIATIONS: Arterioles become narrower; light streak increases to cover more than one third of arteriole; grossly opaque or excessively pale; venules become larger; A-V nicking

Step	Normal/Individual Variations/Deviations
Retinal background for color and surface characteristics	Yellow or pink throughout Fine, granular surface DEVIATIONS: General or localized pallor; hemorrhages of dark or red stains of varying size near vessels; microaneurysms seen as tiny, isolated red dots; drusen
Macular area	Slightly darker than retinal background. Fovea centralis retinae (glistening center point) less bright with advanced age DEVIATION: Increased pigmentation surrounding macula

Sample Documentation—Cataracts

Health History

Mrs. K., 67, reports having more trouble in the last 6 months with blurred vision; adds that she needs a much brighter light and a magnifying glass to read the newspaper. Driving at night has been especially difficult, to the point that she has not done so for about 3 months now, for fear she may have an accident. Denies eye trauma/injury or discharge, excessive or decreased tearing, pain, light flashes, or floaters. No previous eye surgery; no chronic diseases.

Physical Examination

Brows, lids, lashes evenly distributed and equal. No tearing. Conjunctivae pink without discharge. EOMs intact and full, without nystagmus. Visual fields OD decreased temporally and inferiorly. PERRLA. No periorbital edema. No ptosis. Ophthalmoscopic examination reveals a red reflex OS, with creamy pink–colored disc and well-defined border; A-V ratio 2:3 without crossing changes; no hemorrhages or exudates; yellow macula. OD with gray-black reflection; unable to visualize fundus.

Ophthalmoscopic Examination

1. Turn the diaphragm dial so that the small, round white light can be used. Turn on light to maximum brightness (old or defective batteries will reduce lighting).
2. Client should be comfortably seated. Either stand or sit facing the client.
3. Client and examiner remove glasses. Removal of client's contact lenses is optional. It might help to reduce light reflection.
4. Darken the room.
5. Ask the client to hold both eyes open and to direct gaze slightly upward and straight ahead. Gaze should be fixed on some distant object and maintained even if the examiner's head gets in the way.
6. For examination of the client's right eye, hold the ophthalmoscope in your right hand, over your right eye. Stand slightly to the right, at about a 15-degree angle (temporally) from the client.
7. Hold the ophthalmoscope with the index finger on the lens wheel. Rotate the lens wheel to the 0 diopter setting (a lens that neither converges nor diverges light rays).
8. Place your left hand over the client's right eye, with your thumb on the upper brow.
9. Hold the ophthalmoscope firmly against your head and approach to within 30 cm (12 inches) of the client. Direct ophthalmoscope light into the pupil. Continue approach, and red reflex will appear. Try to keep both eyes open.
10. Continue the approach until 3 to 5 cm (1 to 2 inches) from client's eye. Retinal structures should come into view. Clear focus can be established by looking closely at a vessel to see if the borders are sharp. Wheel adjustments need to be made for refractive errors. The myopic client's eyeball may be longer than normal, requir-

Ophthalmoscopic Examination—cont'd

ing rotation of the lens wheel into the red (minus) numbers for clarity. The hyperopic or aphakic client will require lens wheel movement into the black (plus) numbers for clarity.

11. Do not initially focus on the disc. It is helpful to follow vessel bifurcations that lead toward the disc.

12. After inspection of the disc, follow the vessels peripherally in each of four directions. Light must always show *through* the pupil as you inspect in different directions. Beginning examiners often lose their view as they begin to scan the fundus. The client's pupil serves as a stable fulcrum while you and ophthalmoscope move *as a unit* in viewing the retinal periphery.

13. Inspect the retinal background and macula (2 disk diameters [DD] temporal to the disc).

14. After retinal inspection is completed, rotate the lens wheel slowly into the black numbers (0, +5, +10, +15, +20). As the numbers become larger, the anterior surfaces (vitreous, lens) come into view.

15. Slowly rotate the lens wheel up to +20. This should bring the cornea and anterior chamber into focus.

16. Now change to the left eye. Start at client's left, holding the ophthalmoscope with the left hand and over the left eye.

NOTE: Clients who talk during the examination tend to blink and move their eyes more often.

NOTE: Absence of the red reflex may indicate that the eye is abnormal, that the ophthalmoscope is improperly positioned, or that the client has moved his or her eyes. If the red reflex is lost, back away and start over.

NOTE: It is extremely important that you consider your head and the ophthalmoscope as a unit. Be certain that the instrument is stabilized against your brow and cheek.

From Bowers AC, Thompson JM: *Clinical manual of health assessment,* ed 4, St Louis, 1992, Mosby.

Client Teaching

Your Aging Eye

1. Provide bright light when performing tasks such as sewing, reading, and cooking; avoid fluorescent light.
2. Use a magnifying glass if necessary for close work.
3. See your doctor regularly to detect health problems (diabetes, hypertension) that might affect your eyes.
4. Have your eyes examined and a glaucoma test performed every 2 to 3 years by a qualified specialist. Have your eyes examined more frequently if you have a disease or condition that is known to affect vision.
5. Symptoms that require an immediate call to your doctor or eye care specialist include pain, discharge, redness or swelling, and loss of vision, no matter how slight.
6. Artificial tears may relieve dry eyes, which is a common condition. Check with your health care practitioner before using any such over-the-counter preparation.
7. Excessive tearing can be a benign condition or it may reflect a more serious problem. See your health care practitioner or eye care specialist if you are troubled by this problem.
8. Floaters, a common occurrence in older persons, are just spots or flecks that literally "float" across your field of vision. They usually occur gradually and are most noticeable in a brightly lit environment. If they occur in association with light flashes in your visual field, call your health care practitioner or eye care specialist.
9. Cataracts are a normal part of the aging process that develop gradually and without pain. When tasks become increasingly more difficult and fatiguing, however, because of the vision changes cataracts produce, see your health care practitioner or eye care specialist to discuss treatment options.

Compiled from *Aging and your eyes.* (1991). Age Page, National Institute on Aging, Bethesda, Md, US Department of Health and Human Services, Public Health Service, National Institutes of Health.

References

Aging and your eyes, Age Page, National Institute on Aging, Bethesda, Md, 1991, US Department of Health and Human Services, Public Health Service, National Institutes of Health.

Barkauskas VH et al: *Health and physical assessment,* ed 2, St Louis, 1998, Mosby.

Bowers AC, Thompson JM: *Clinical manual of health assessment,* ed 4, St Louis, 1992, Mosby.

Malasanos L et al: *Health assessment,* ed 4, St Louis, 1990, Mosby.

Thibodeau GA, Patton KT: *Anatomy and physiology,* ed 3, St Louis, 1996, Mosby.

Thompson JM, Bowers AC: *Health assessment: an illustrated pocket guide,* ed 3, St Louis, 1992, Mosby.

Assessment of the Ears, Nose, and Throat

9

Assessment of the ears, nose, and throat provides data about the upper respiratory system and the beginning of the digestive system. Valuable information about problems specific to these areas and information about overall health can be obtained. The skills of inspection and palpation are used. Equipment needs include an otoscope with specula, olfactory and taste testing substances, watch, tongue blade, gauze sponges, gloves, tuning fork with frequencies of 500 to 1000 cps, penlight, and cerumen spoon.

Anatomy and Physiology

Ear

The ear, as the organ of hearing and equilibrium, contains receptors that convert sound waves into nerve impulses and receptors that respond to movements of the head. The ear is divided into three parts: external, middle, and inner ear (Fig. 9-1).

The external ear consists of the auricle, or pinna, and the external auditory canal. The function of the external ear is to perceive sound. The auricle is composed mostly of cartilage covered with skin. Its main components are the helix, antihelix, antitragus, lobule, tragus, concha, and triangular fossa (Fig. 9-2). The lobe is the only portion not supported with cartilage. As a person ages, cartilage continues to be formed in the ears, and the skin of the ears loses elasticity; thus the auricle appears larger and the lobule is elongated. Accompanying these age-related changes is wrinkling

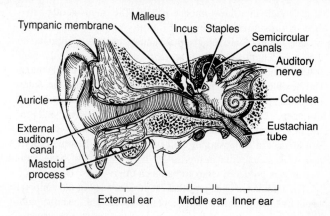

Fig. 9-1
Ear structures. (From Potter PA: *Pocket guide to health assessment,*
ed 3, St Louis, 1994, Mosby.)

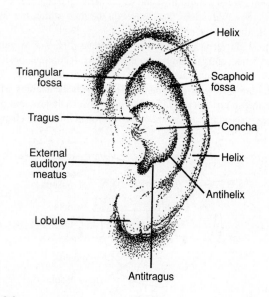

Fig. 9-2
Anatomic structures of the human ear, with features of aging.
(From Thompson JM et al: *Mosby's manual of clinical nursing,* ed 3,
St Louis, 1993, Mosby.)

of the lobule in a linear oblique pattern. The tragus is often covered by tufts of coarse hair.

The slightly S-shaped external auditory canal is approximately 2.5 cm in length and extends upward from the auricle to the tympanic membrane. The distal portion of the canal is cartilaginous and flexible; the inner portion is bony and fixed. The skin lining the canal near the entrance contains cilia and sebaceous glands. Cerumen secreted by the glands captures foreign material and protects the canal epithelium. With aging, the canal narrows as a result of inward collapsing of the canal wall. Cilia become coarser and stiffer, and cerumen production decreases slightly; the cerumen that is produced tends to be much drier.

The middle ear is an air-filled chamber located in the temporal bone. Its function is to amplify captured sound. This chamber contains three articulating ossicles—the malleus, incus, and stapes—that are attached to the wall of the tympanic chamber by ligaments. The tympanic membrane separates the middle ear from the external auditory canal. Vibrations of the membrane cause the ossicles to move and transmit sound waves across the chamber to the oval window. Vibrations then move via the fluid within the inner ear and stimulate hearing receptors.

The slightly concave tympanic membrane (Fig. 9-3) is pulled inward at its center, or umbo, by the malleus. Its oblique position to the canal accounts for the cone of light, or light reflex. The dense, fibrous ring surrounding the membrane is the annulus. Most of the membrane is taut, called the pars tensa. The less taut pars flaccida is the superior portion of the membrane. Atrophic changes

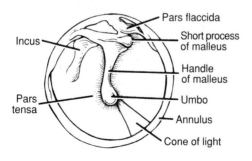

Fig. 9-3
Normal tympanic membrane. (From Potter PA: *Pocket guide to health assessment,* ed 3, St Louis, 1994, Mosby.)

in the membrane caused by aging result in a dull, retracted, white or gray appearance. These changes have no apparent effect on hearing.

The inner ear, or labyrinth, contains the functional organs for hearing and equilibrium. The inner ear consists of two parts: the outer bony labyrinth and the membranous labyrinth within the bony labyrinth. The bony labyrinth is structurally and functionally divided into three areas: vestibule, semicircular canals, and cochlea. The vestibule and semicircular canals contain receptors for equilibrium. The cochlea is a coiled structure containing the organ of Corti, the functional unit of hearing (Fig. 9-1). Hair cells of the organ of Corti are bent or distorted by vibrations entering the cochlea, which are then converted into electrochemical impulses. Degenerative changes in the cochlea and neurons of higher auditory pathways result in presbycusis, a bilateral, progressive, sensorineural hearing loss that begins in middle age. The ability to hear high-frequency sounds is affected first, followed by sounds in the middle range, then low-frequency sounds.

Nose and Nasal Cavity

The nasal cavity's functions are to warm, filter, and moisten incoming air and to identify odors. The nose is divided into the external nose and the nasal cavity. The external nose is covered with skin; it is supported by paired nasal bones, which form the bridge, and by pliable cartilage, which forms the distal portions. The nasal septum divides the nasal cavity into halves, each called a nasal fossa. Each fossa opens anteriorly through the nostrils, or nares, and posteriorly through the choanae, or posterior nares. The roof of the nasal cavity is formed anteriorly by the frontal bone and paired nasal bones, medially by a portion of the ethmoid bone, and posteriorly by the sphenoid bone (Fig. 9-4). The floor of the cavity is formed by the palatine and maxillary bones. The lateral walls consist of the superior, middle, and inferior turbinate bones, which protrude into the nasal cavity and are covered by a highly vascular mucous membrane. The space below each turbinate is a meatus, named for the turbinate above it. The nasolacrimal duct drains tears from the eye into the inferior meatus. Most of the paranasal sinuses drain into the medial meatus. Receptors for the olfactory nerve (CN I) lie on the upper third of the nasal septum. These receptor cells pass through holes in the ethmoid bone to the olfactory bulb, then to the temporal lobe of the brain, where impulses are interpreted as smell. Cartilage continues to form in the nose with

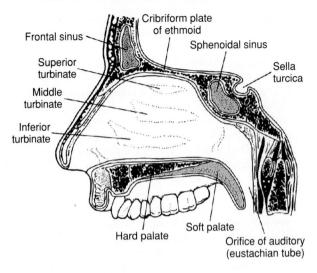

Fig. 9-4
Sagittal section of the nose. (Redrawn from Seidel HM et al: *Mosby's guide to physical examination,* ed 3, St Louis, 1995, Mosby.)

aging, causing the nose to protrude more sharply. Progressive atrophy of the olfactory bulbs also occurs, resulting in a gradual decline in the sense of smell.

The paranasal sinuses are paired air spaces in certain facial bones. There are the maxillary, frontal, sphenoidal, and ethmoidal sinuses (Fig. 9-5). Each sinus communicates via drainage ducts within the nasal cavity on the side where it is located.

Mouth and Oropharynx

The functions of the mouth and associated structures are to serve as a receptacle for food, to initiate digestion through mastication, to swallow food, to form words in speech, and to identify taste. The mouth also serves as a passageway for air. The structures of the mouth include the lips, hard and soft palate, tongue, teeth and gums, and salivary glands (Fig. 9-6).

The lips form the anterior border of the mouth and have the principal function of facilitating speech. Sensory receptors in the lips aid in determining texture and temperature of food.

The roof of the mouth is formed by the white hard palate ante-

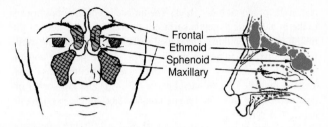

Fig. 9-5
Location of sinuses. (From Phipps WJ et al: *Medical-surgical nursing,* ed 5, St Louis, 1993, Mosby.)

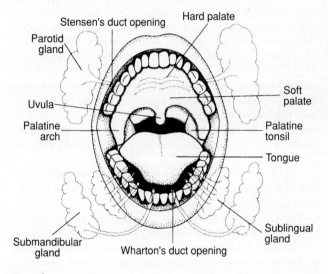

Fig. 9-6
Structures of the mouth. (Redrawn from Malasanos L et al: *Health assessment,* ed 4, St Louis, 1990, Mosby.)

riorly and the pink soft palate posteriorly. The uvula is suspended from the middle lower border of the soft palate. During swallowing, both the uvula and soft palate are forced upward, closing the nasopharynx and preventing food and fluid from entering the nasal cavity.

The tongue assists in the mastication and swallowing of food and in the production of speech. The tongue is attached posteriorly to the hyoid bone; the undersurface is connected to the floor of the mouth by the frenulum. The dorsal surface has many small papillae that give the tongue a rough texture. These papillae contain taste buds that distinguish sweet, salty, sour, and bitter sensations. Taste is mediated by the facial nerve (CN VII) and glossopharyngeal nerve (CN IX). The tongue is innervated by the hypoglossal nerve (CN XII).

The gums, or gingivae, consist of fibrous tissue covered with mucus membrane; they blanket the bony ridges of the mandible and maxilla as well as the necks of the teeth. Adults have 32 teeth, 16 in each arch (Fig. 9-7).

Three pairs of salivary glands secrete into the oral cavity: parotid, submandibular, and sublingual. Saliva functions as a solvent in cleansing teeth and dissolving food chemicals for tasting. Enzymes in saliva digest starch, and mucus provides lubrication. The parotid gland is the largest and lies just below and in front of the ear. The parotid (Stensen's) duct drains into the oral cavity opposite the second upper molar. The submandibular (Wharton's) duct empties into the floor of the mouth on either side of the frenulum. The sublingual glands are the smallest; they are located on the floor of the mouth between the sides of the tongue and the mandible. Each of these glands has many small openings along the sublingual fold.

The oropharynx extends from the soft palate to the epiglottis. The base of the tongue forms its anterior wall. The tonsils are located on the posterior lateral walls.

The mouth and oropharynx show many changes with advancing age. Tooth enamel is abraded, and underlying dentin thickens, which results in yellowing of the teeth. Tooth surfaces wear down from long use. Gums recede, exposing the tooth root. Taste buds decrease in number, so taste perception is altered. Salivary secretion is reduced because of degeneration of the epithelial lining of the glands, and saliva becomes more mucoid and thicker.

Periodontal structures (the gingivae, alveolar bone, periodontal membrane, and cementum) become ischemic and undergo fibrotic changes. Osteoblasts and fibroblasts are less active, so they are slow to repair daily wear and tear. Consequently, periodontal structures of older adults atrophy and degenerate more easily than those of younger people; this can lead to loss of teeth.

Bacterial plaque in clients over 50 is usually produced by

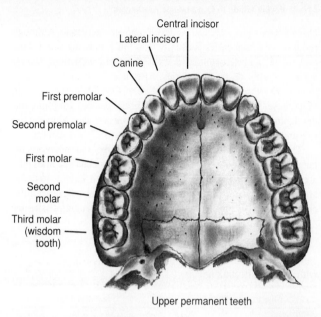

Upper permanent teeth

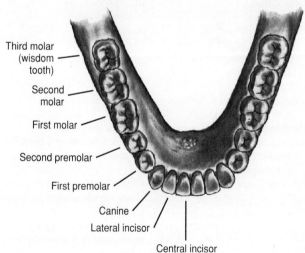

Lower permanent teeth

Fig. 9-7
Dentition of permanent teeth. (Adapted from Seidel HM et al: *Mosby's guide to physical examination,* ed 3, St. Louis, 1995, Mosby.)

Odontomyces viscosus. Caries develop under the plaque. Although progress of dental caries is usually slow, older persons with friable oral tissues and xerostomia (decreased saliva production) rapidly develop highly destructive caries. After age 70, bacterial populations of *O. viscosus* decrease and those of *Candida albicans* begin to increase. The characteristic white, cheesy patches are found under dentures and along the cheek and tongue surfaces. Mucosal tissue underneath the candida infection is raw, red, and painful.

The overall increase in tissue friability of the oral mucosa is related to three separate sources. First, the oral mucosa becomes progressively drier as a consequence of diminished kidney function and a shift in water balance from the intracellular to extracellular compartment. Second, the epithelial layer thins, leaving tissue un-

Table 9-1   Systemic diseases and conditions associated with oral manifestations

Disease/Condition	Manifestation
Osteoporosis	Resorption of the mandibular alveolar ridge
Diabetes mellitus, diabetes insipidus, nephritis, drug therapy, pernicious anemia, and irradiation	Xerostomia
Liver cirrhosis	Oral cancer
Vitamin A, B, and C deficiencies	Periodontal disease
	Glossitis
Antibiotic therapy	*Candida* infection
Vitamin A deficiency, anemias, chronic fever, and vitamin B deficiencies	Tongue fissuring and depapillation
Emotional stress	Canker sores, traumatic ulcers, angular cheilosis
Malnutrition	Cheilosis
	Swollen, smooth tongue
	Hyperemic and hypertrophic papillae
	Spongy, bleeding, receding gums
	Cracked, crusted, tender lips

protected and thus vulnerable, even to minor stresses. Third, mucosal cells are usually undernourished, resulting in reduced tissue resistance to injury and infection.

The height and width of the alveolar ridge gradually decrease as a result of bone resorption, particularly in edentulous persons who wear dentures. Xerostomia can result from systemic illness (diabetes mellitus, diabetes insipidus, nephritis, pernicious anemia), drugs (phenothiazines, antidepressants, antiparkinsonian agents, *Rauwolfia* derivatives, anticholinergics), and conditions such as vitamin deficiencies and effects of irradiation (Table 9-1).

Assessment of the Ears

Equipment needed:
    Otoscope with specula
    Watch with audible tick
    Tuning fork with frequency of 500 to 1000 cps
    Cerumen spoon

Step	Normal/Individual Variations/Deviations
With client sitting, inspect auricles for position, size, and symmetry	Top of pinna level with corner of the eye; pinna no more than 10 degrees off vertical line
	Ears of equal height and size with symmetric placement
	Earlobes may be elongated
	DEVIATIONS: Unequal positioning, size; low set

NOTE: The above screening tests are crude measures; clients demonstrating hearing loss by screening should be referred to a specialist for comprehensive audiologic evaluation. See the box on p. 175.   *Continued*

Step	Normal/Individual Variations/Deviations
Palpate auricles and mastoid for swelling, tenderness, and nodules	Firm, mobile, nontender, without nodules DEVIATIONS: Tenderness, pain, swelling, nodules; tophi; lesions
Assess internal structures with the otoscope (see the box on p. 171)	
Auditory canal for cerumen, foreign objects, lesions, and discharge	Cerumen yellow to brown or black in color; moist to flaky or hard texture Free of foreign objects, lesions, or discharge; coarse hair may be present at entrance DEVIATIONS: Impacted cerumen; presence of foreign objects, lesions, or discharge; pain, tenderness, swelling
Tympanic membrane for color and landmarks	Translucent, shiny, pearly gray membrane; may be dull, white Landmarks of umbo, malleus, cone of light, anulus, pars tensa, and pars flaccida visible; may appear slightly more pronounced from sclerotic changes DEVIATIONS: Amber, blue, or pink to red in color; bulging membrane with loss of landmarks and distorted cone of light; retracted membrane with accentuated landmarks and distorted cone of light

NOTE: The above screening tests are crude measures; clients demonstrating hearing loss by screening should be referred to a specialist for comprehensive audiologic evaluation. See the box on p. 175.

Step	Normal/Individual Variations/Deviations
Assess auditory function (CN VIII) by performing screening hearing tests:	
Voice test	Able to hear softly whispered words with 50% accuracy at distance of 1 to 2 feet in both ears
Technique: With opposite ear occluded, stand 1 to 2 feet from ear being tested. While standing behind client to prevent lip-reading, softly whisper numbers and ask client to repeat. Gradually increase intensity of whisper until client correctly repeats with 50% accuracy. Repeat steps with other ear.	DEVIATIONS: Unable to accurately repeat until voice is louder; bilaterally unequal response
Watch-tick test	Able to hear ticking watch at distance of 1 to 2 inches
Technique: With opposite ear occluded, place ticking watch about 5 inches from ear, slowly moving watch toward the ear. Ask client to indicate when ticking is heard. Repeat steps with other ear.	Wide range of variation in distance depending on degree of presbycusis. DEVIATIONS: Unable to hear ticking
Tuning fork (Weber test)	Bilaterally equal sound
Technique: Place vibrating tuning fork on client's forehead. Instruct client to indicate if sound is heard equally in both ears or better in one ear (lateralization of sound).	May have some degree of perceptive loss (presbycusis). DEVIATIONS: Conductive loss lateralized to poorer ear; marked sensorineural or perceptive loss lateralized to better ear (Table 9-2)

Continued

Step	Normal/Individual Variations/Deviations
Tuning fork (Rinne test) **Technique:** Place vibrating tuning fork against mastoid bone and begin noting time in seconds. Instruct client to indicate when sound is no longer heard; note time lapsed in seconds. Quickly move still vibrating fork 1 inch from auditory canal and again instruct client to indicate when sound is no longer heard. Continue noting time elapsed in seconds until sound is no longer heard. Repeat steps with other ear.	Air conduction (AC) approximately twice as long as bone conduction (BC); (AC > BC) DEVIATIONS: BC > AC, indicative of hearing loss; air conduction heard longer but not twice as long as bone conduction, indicative of sensorineural loss (Table 9-2)

NOTE: The above screening tests are crude measures; clients demonstrating hearing loss by screening should be referred to a specialist for comprehensive audiologic evaluation. See the box on p. 175.

Assessment of the Nose and Nasal Cavity

Equipment needed:
   Otoscope with specula or nasal speculum
   Olfactory testing substances

Step	Normal/Individual Variations/Deviations
With client sitting, inspect	
External nose for shape, size, and color	Symmetric or nearly symmetric alignment
	Color consistent with that of face
	DEVIATIONS: Gross asymmetry; bulbous appearance; redness or other discoloration; increased vascularization
Nares for symmetry, flaring, discharge	Symmetric, without flaring or discharge; dry without crusting
	DEVIATIONS: Grossly asymmetric; flaring associated with breathing; discharge present; crusting
Nares for patency	Bilaterally equal free exchange of air
Technique: Occlude one naris by pressing finger on side of nose. Instruct client to breathe in and out with mouth closed. Hold finger under open naris, and note air flow. Repeat steps with other side.	DEVIATIONS: Unequal response (alerts examiner to assess for possible occlusion on internal examination)

Continued

Step	Normal/Individual Variations/Deviations
Assess olfactory function (CN I)	Able to identify strong odors
Technique: Have available two vials of familiar, fragrant odors (coffee, cloves, peppermint). Instruct client to close eyes while you occlude one naris and hold open vial under nose. Have client breathe deeply through open naris and identify odor. Repeat with other side; after brief rest period, repeat entire procedure with second odor.	DEVIATIONS: Unable to identify strong odors
Assess internal cavity with otoscope	
Technique: With right hand covering forehead and top of head to control client's position, hold otoscope in left hand with index finger placed on side of nose to stabilize position of speculum and prevent displacement. Insert speculum slowly and cautiously.	

Step	Normal/Individual Variations/Deviations
With client's head erect, inspect	
Mucosa for color, discharge, masses, lesions	Pink, moist appearing, covered with clear mucus
	No crusting, masses, or lesions
	DEVIATIONS: Fiery red or pale gray; crusting, discharge, masses, lesions
Septum for alignment, perforation, bleeding, crusting	Septum divides nasal cavity into two equal chambers
	No perforations, bleeding, or crusting
	DEVIATIONS: Masses, bleeding, or crusting; septal perforation or deviation
Inferior turbinate	No swelling, polyps, or lesions
	DEVIATIONS: Swelling, polyps, or lesions; pale
Continuing with client's head tilted back:	
Inspect middle turbinate	As described above
	DEVIATIONS: As described above
Palpate frontal and maxillary sinuses for tenderness	Nontender
	DEVIATIONS: Tender
Technique: Press thumbs firmly under bony brow on each side of nose (frontal), then under the zygomatic processes (maxillary). Fingers of both hands should be placed over lateral head to stabilize while exerting pressure with thumbs.	

Assessment of the Mouth and Oropharynx

Equipment needed:
  Penlight
  Tongue blade
  Gauze sponges
  Gloves
  Taste testing substances

Step	Normal/Individual Variations/Deviations
Inspect Lips for shape, position, movement, condition, color, lesions	Vertical and horizontal symmetry at rest and with facial movement No cracks or fissures, but increased vertical markings; may be dry; pink to brown without lesions DEVIATIONS: Swelling; deep fissures at corner of mouth; cracked; pale, reddened, or cyanotic; plaques, vesicles, nodules, or ulcerations
Buccal mucosa for color, texture, lesions	Pink, smooth, moist May appear less vascular and shiny Fordyce's spots common DEVIATIONS: Pale, reddened or cyanotic; white or gray patches; ulcers, swelling, bleeding
Gums for color and surface characteristics	Pink to pale in color Clearly defined, tight margin at tooth DEVIATIONS: Bright red or markedly pale; retracted, bleeding, discolored; enlarged crevices between teeth and gum margins

Step	Normal/Individual Variations/Deviations
Teeth for occlusion, number, color, and surface characteristics	Top back teeth rest on lower teeth; upper incisors slightly override lowers
	Thirty-two full adult teeth; some may be missing depending on history
	Yellow or grayer in color
	May be worn down or appear longer
	DEVIATIONS: Malocclusion; several teeth missing, darkened or stained, loose or broken teeth; deteriorated dental restorations
Tongue for color, texture, size, coating, or ulcerations	Pink, smooth appearance
	Fits easily into mouth
	Moist to slightly dry but glistening
	No lesions
	DEVIATIONS: Beefy red; nodules or areas of induration present; deep furrowing, swelling; markedly smooth surface; lesions
Assess hypoglossal function (CN XII)	Symmetric appearance, lies in midline
Technique: Instruct client to rest tongue on floor of mouth. Note movement and symmetry.	DEVIATIONS: Fasciculations, asymmetry, atrophy, or deviation from midline
Instruct client to stick out tongue and move from side to side, curl upward, and curl downward.	Smooth, even movement of tongue
	DEVIATIONS: Slow alternate movements; tongue deviates to one side
Instruct client to repeat a phrase containing words with the letters *l, t, d,* or *n.*	Crisp, clear articulation of sounds; words intact
	DEVIATIONS: Unclear articulation of sounds

Continued

Step	Normal/Individual Variations/Deviations
Inspect	
Floor of mouth for color, surface characteristics	Pink without lesions or masses DEVIATIONS: Pale or reddened; varicosities, swelling
Hard and soft palate for color, contour, and movement	Soft palate pink, hard palate whiter; may have bony protuberance at midline (torus palatinus) Gently, smoothly, symmetrically arched DEVIATIONS: Pale or reddened; high or pointed arch
Tonsillar areas for size, color, exudate	Tonsils may be cryptic; symmetric and without swelling Pink to pale without exudate DEVIATIONS: Hypertrophied; reddened; crypts with exudate or debris
Posterior pharyngeal wall for color, discharge, lesions	Pink to pale without discharge or lesions DEVIATIONS: Reddened with exudate
Assess glossopharyngeal (CN IX) and vagus (CN X) nerves **Technique:** Instruct client to say "ahh." **Technique:** Gently touch posterior wall of pharynx with tongue blade, then quickly withdraw.	Soft palate elevates symmetrically; uvula rises at midline DEVIATIONS: Unilateral elevation, deviation of uvula Gag will occur DEVIATIONS: No gag reflex

Step	Normal/Individual Variations/Deviations
Palpate tongue and floor of mouth for tenderness, masses **Technique:** Wearing gloves, palpate tongue between thumb and forefinger; palpate floor with index finger.	Nontender without swelling, masses, or ulcerations DEVIATIONS: Tenderness; ulcerations, nodules, or thickening
Assess facial (CN VII) and glossopharyngeal (CN IX) function **Technique:** Have available bitter, sour, salty, and sweet solutions, applicators, and a card listing the tastes. Apply one solution at a time to the lateral side of the tongue on the following regions: Bitter—extreme posterior third Sour—near middle Salty—posterior region of anterior two thirds Sweet—lateral tip Have client keep tongue protruded and point to taste on card that describes solution tasted. Give client a sip of water between solutions. Test both sides of tongue.	Able to identify each taste bilaterally; reduced taste perception overall, especially sweet and salty tastes DEVIATIONS: Unable to identify tastes unilaterally or bilaterally

Sample Documentation—Sinusitis

Health History

Mrs. J., 72, reports 2-day duration of pain around both eyes, yellow nasal discharge, and generally feeling "lousy." Ears feel "stuffy," and upper teeth hurt. Denies fever, chills, sore throat, cough.

Physical Examination

Bilateral periorbital edema and dark skin noted below eyes. Bilateral frontal and maxillary sinus pain elicited on light palpation. Moderate amount of yellow, purulent rhinorrhea in nasal cavities, with bright red, turgescent mucosa; purulent exudate also noted in meatus of middle turbinate. Pharynx without redness or exudate. Ear canals unobstructed with small amount of amber cerumen AU. TMs intact with light reflex and bony landmarks present, but with sclerotic changes noted.

The screening questionnaire on p. 175 is a useful tool for screening both communication problems and the social and emotional disabilities associated with hearing loss. This instrument has been found to have sensitivity and specificity values between 60% and 80%—not quite as high as the values for audiometry screening. Therefore some authorities recommend using both a questionnaire of this type and pure-tone testing for screening purposes, which may improve sensitivity and specificity.

Otoscopic Examination Guidelines

1. Use the largest speculum that will fit comfortably into the ear canal.
2. The otoscope must have good batteries or adequate illumination of the landmarks of the ear will be impossible. (Batteries should give off white, *not* yellow, light.)
3. The adult client should be sitting with the head tilted toward the opposite shoulder.
4. Hold the otoscope between the palm and the first two fingers of one hand. The handle may be positioned either downward or upward. Determine which position provides better immobility between the otoscope and the client's head.
5. With the other hand, grasp the pinna with the thumb and fingers and pull out, up, and back to straighten the canal.
6. Remember, the inner two thirds of the external ear canal are bony. It will *hurt* if the speculum is pressed against either side. If you are having difficulty seeing the tympanic membrane, attempt a combination of repositioning the head, pulling the auricle in a slightly different position, and reangling the otoscope.
7. When placing the speculum in the client's ear, make sure to steady your hand against the client's head by extending one or two fingers from the hand holding the otoscope.

From Bowers AC, Thompson JM: *Clinical manual of health assessment,* ed 4, St Louis, 1992, Mosby.

Table 9-2 Hearing tests using tuning fork

Hearing	Weber (Bone Conduction)	Rinne (Air and Bone Conduction)
Normal	**Normal hearing** Sound is heard equally well in both ears; no lateralization	**Normal hearing** Sound is heard twice as long by air conduction (AC) as by bone conduction (BC); AC:BC 2:1

Conduction loss
(problem of
external or
middle ear,
e.g., cerumen
buildup or
otitis media)

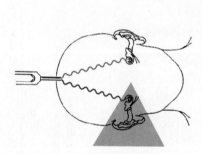

Conductive deafness
Sound lateralizes to defective ear because it is
transmitted through bone rather than air

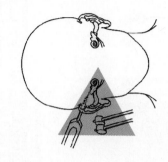

Conductive deafness
Sound is heard longer by bone conduction than
by air conduction; BC > AC

Continued

Table 9-2   Hearing tests using tuning fork—cont'd

Hearing	Weber (Bone Conduction)	Rinne (Air and Bone Conduction)

Sensorineural loss (perceptive problem of inner ear or nerve)

Perceptive deafness
Sound lateralizes to better ear

Perceptive deafness
Sound is heard longer by air conduction than by bone conduction (AC > BC) but for a shorter duration than with normal hearing

From Barkauskas VH et al: *Health and physical assessment*, St Louis, 1994, Mosby.

Hearing Disability Inventory in the Elderly Screening Questionnaire

Instructions: Check one answer for each question. Do not skip a question if you avoid a situation because of a hearing problem. If you use a hearing aid, please answer according to the way you hear without the aid.

Question	Yes	No	Sometimes	
1. Does a hearing problem cause you to feel embarrassed when you meet new people?				
2. Does a hearing problem cause you to feel frustrated when talking to members of your family?				
3. Do you have difficulty hearing when someone speaks in a whisper?				
4. Do you feel disabled by a hearing problem?				
5. Does a hearing problem cause you difficulty when visiting friends, relatives, or neighbors?				
6. Does a hearing problem cause you to attend religious services less often than you would like?				
7. Does a hearing problem cause you to have arguments with family members?				
8. Does a hearing problem cause you difficulty when listening to TV or radio?				
9. Do you feel that any difficulty with your hearing limits or hampers your personal or social life?				
10. Does a hearing problem cause you difficulty when in a restaurant with relatives or friends?				

Scoring: No = 0; Sometimes = 2; Yes = 4.
Interpretation of total scores: 0-8 = no disability; 10-24 = mild to moderate disability; 26-40 = severe disability.

Adapted from Ventry I, Weinstein B. Identification of elderly people with hearing problems, *ASHA,* 25:37-42, 1983. Reproduced by permission of the American Speech and Hearing Association; © 1983. From Adult screening for hearing, *Nurse Pract* 21:106, 108, 115, 1996.

Client Teaching

Hearing Loss

1. Presbycusis is the normal hearing loss associated with aging. Changes in the structure and function of the inner ear make it difficult to understand certain types of speech sounds and produce an intolerance for loud noise. The sounds that are usually lost first are *f, s, th, ch,* and *sh.* As hearing loss progresses, the ability to hear the sounds of *b, t, p, k,* and *t* is also impaired.
2. Some of the most common signs and symptoms of hearing loss include the following:
   a. Difficulty understanding speech
   b. Inability to hear high-pitched sounds
   c. Difficulty discriminating speech; another person's speech sounds slurred or mumbled
   d. Trouble hearing at large gatherings, especially where there is background noise
   e. A constant ringing or hissing background noise
3. Do not be afraid to tell family and friends to face you and to speak at a normal rate, in lower tones (not necessarily louder), and with greater clarity. If you do not understand, ask the person to repeat. Listen carefully while watching the person's face and lips.
4. If you are having a hearing problem, see your health care practitioner. A hearing problem may be caused by a serious medical condition that your health care practitioner may be able to diagnose and treat, or your health care practitioner may wish to refer you to a specialist for further evaluation.
5. A hearing aid may be recommended. Seek professional guidance in obtaining the best aid suited to your specific needs. Find a reputable dealer by checking with the Better Business Bureau. Because of the high cost of hearing aids and their upkeep, it is wise to choose carefully.

Compiled from *Hearing and older people,* Age Page, National Institute on Aging, Bethesda, Md, 1991, US Department of Health and Human Services, Public Health Service, National Institutes of Health.

Client Teaching—cont'd

Oral Health Care

1. Preventive oral care is a lifelong requirement, even for denture wearers. See your dentist regularly for care and treatment.
2. Periodontal disease is the most common cause of tooth loss after age 35 years. It is caused by the buildup of plaque. The bacteria in plaque irritate the gums, causing inflammation and bleeding. If plaque is not removed, infection forms between the teeth and gums, creating gum recession. The infection spreads to the roots of the teeth, eventually causing tooth loss. Common signs and symptoms of periodontal disease include the following:
   a. Red, swollen, and/or bleeding gums
   b. Sensitive and/or painful gums
   c. Pus between gums and teeth
   d. Receding gums
   e. Loose teeth
3. Measures for preventing periodontal disease include the following:
   a. Brushing teeth at least daily, preferably after every meal. Using a soft-bristle brush and fluoride toothpaste, brush with circular, short back-and-forth motions, paying special attention to the gum line itself.
   b. Flossing daily to remove plaque and other food debris that brushing does not reach. If flossing causes gum irritation or bleeding on an ongoing basis, see your dentist as soon as possible.
   c. Using an antibacterial or antiplaque mouth rinse. Your dentist can suggest one for you.
4. Oral hygiene practices should not stop with the loss of natural teeth. Care of dentures and the mouth structures is important for overall health and comfort. Food, stains, and tartar can collect on dentures too. Mouth care for persons with dentures includes the following:
   a. Brushing at least daily, preferably after every meal. Food debris caught between the palate and denture can cause traumatic injury to the mouth tissue.

Continued

Client Teaching—cont'd

    b. Removing dentures each night and placing in water or a denture-cleaning solution to prevent drying or warping of the dentures.

    c. Rinsing mouth with warm water before replacing dentures in the morning, after meals, and at bedtime.

5. See your dentist if any of the following occur in your mouth:

    a. Sores that bleed, or red or white spots that do not go away within 2 weeks.

    b. Pain anywhere in your mouth.

6. Dry mouth is a common occurrence that could result from decreased salivary gland function or medication side effect. A chronically dry mouth can promote tooth decay and gum disease, so see your dentist or doctor for treatment. To relieve the dryness, drink water regularly and avoid sugary foods and snacks, caffeinated drinks, alcohol, and tobacco.

Compiled from *Hearing and older people,* Age Page, National Institute on Aging, Bethesda, Md, 1991, US Department of Health and Human Services, Public Health Service, National Institutes of Health.

References

Barkauskas VH et al: *Health and physical assessment,* ed 2, St Louis, 1998, Mosby.

Bowers AC, Thompson JM: *Clinical manual of health assessment,* ed 4, St Louis, 1992, Mosby.

Hearing and older people, Age Page, National Institute on Aging, Bethesda, Md, 1991, US Department of Health and Human Services, Public Health Service, National Institutes of Health.

Malasanos L et al: *Health assessment,* ed 4, St Louis, 1990, Mosby.

Phipps WJ et al: *Medical-surgical nursing,* ed 5, St Louis, 1995, Mosby.

Potter PA: *Pocket guide to health assessment,* ed 3, St Louis, 1994, Mosby.

Seidel HM et al: *Mosby's guide to physical examination,* ed 3, St Louis, 1995, Mosby.

Thompson JM et al: *Mosby's manual of clinical nursing,* ed 3, St Louis, 1993, Mosby.

Clinical guidelines: adult screening for hearing, *Nurse Pract* 21:106, 108, 115, 1996.

Assessment of the Breasts

10

Assessment of the breasts involves the actual structures of each breast as well as the axillae. The axillae are clinically important because the lymphatics of most of the breast drain toward this area. The breasts of both males and females should be examined; male breast enlargement, or gynecomastia, may normally occur in older males. Inspection and palpation are the skills used in breast examination. A centimeter ruler may be necessary to measure location and size of lesions or masses. A small pillow or towel is used when examining the breast of the client in the supine position.

Anatomy and Physiology

Breasts and Mammary Glands

The breasts are located on the anterior chest wall between the second and sixth ribs, overlying the pectoralis major muscle and portions of the serratus anterior and external oblique muscles. The medial boundary is the lateral margin of the sternum, and the lateral boundary is the anterior axillary line. The axillary tail, or tail of Spence, extends upward and laterally toward the axilla. The breast is supported by a layer of subcutaneous connective tissue and fat. Cooper's suspensory ligaments are fibrous bands that extend from the connective tissue layer through the breasts, attaching to the muscle fascia (Fig. 10-1, *B*).

The mammary glands within the breasts are actually modified sweat glands. Each gland consists of 15 to 20 lobes divided by adipose tissue. Each lobe is divided into 20 to 40 lobules that contain the acini cells. Milk produced in these cells is secreted into tubules that converge into lactiferous ducts. These ducts drain milk out through the nipple (Fig. 10-1, *A*).

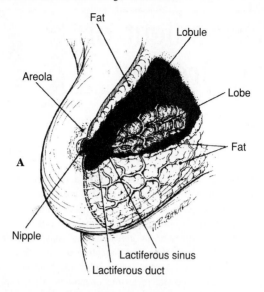

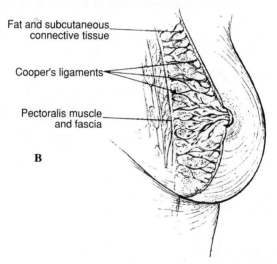

Fig. 10-1
Female breasts **A,** Supportive tissue structures. **B,** Internal structures. (From Malasanos L et al: *Health assessment,* ed 4, St Louis, 1990, Mosby.)

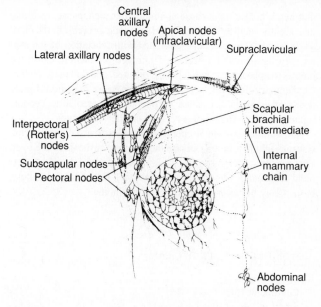

Fig. 10-2

Lymphatic drainage of breast. (Modified from Thompson JM: *Clinical outlines for health assessment,* St Louis, 1997, Mosby.)

The nipple is a round, protuberant structure surrounded by the areola, located at the center of the breast. The pigmentation of the nipple and areola varies greatly. Some hair follicles may be present around the areola.

Lymphatics

The lymphatic system of each breast consists of three types of lymphatics: cutaneous, deep, and areolar. Cutaneous lymphatics drain the skin of the breast into the scapular, brachial, and intermediate nodes toward the axillary nodes and into the lateral mammary chain. Deep lymphatics drain the deep mammary tissues into the subscapular, pectoral, interpectoral, and brachial, or lateral axillary nodes. Areolar lymphatics drain the areolar and nipple areas of the breast into the mammary, apical, and supraclavicular nodes (Fig. 10-2).

The atrophy of glandular tissue and increase in adipose tissue that begin before menopause continue after menopause, resulting in a slightly smaller, less dense, and less nodular breast in the older adult female. These changes, coupled with relaxation of the suspensory ligaments and decreased estrogen production, cause the breasts to appear more pendulous, elongated, and flattened. The inframammary ridge thickens, allowing for easier palpation. Lower levels of estrogen also cause the nipples and areolae to become lighter in color. The nipples become smaller and flatter.

Gynecomastia in men after age 50 years is usually unilateral. Causes include testicular or pituitary tumors, cirrhosis of the liver, estrogen drug therapy for prostatic cancer, and therapy with steroidal compounds (digitalis, spironolactone). Depending on history, biopsy may be necessary to rule out carcinoma.

Assessment of the Breasts

Equipment needed:
  Centimeter ruler
  Small pillow or towel

Step	Normal/Individual Variations/Deviations
With client sitting upright, disrobed to waist, arms at sides, inspect	
Breasts for size and symmetry, contour, skin color and texture, venous patterns, and lesions	Wide variation of size, usually asymmetric
	Smooth, uninterrupted contour; pendulous, flabby and flattened; low hanging on chest wall
	Even color consistent with overall body pigmentation; smooth texture
	Venous patterns similar bilaterally
	Unchanged, nontender, long-standing lesions

Figures shown on pp. 183-186 from Malasanos L et al: *Health assessment,* ed 4, St Louis, 1990, Mosby.

Step	Normal/Individual Variations/Deviations

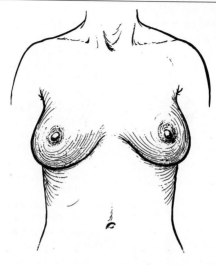

DEVIATIONS: Client report of recent increase in size or gross asymmetry; retractions, dimpling, bulging; redness, hyperpigmentation; thickening, edema *(peau d'orange);* unilateral venous patterns or increased venous prominence; change in or recent onset of any lesions

Areolae for size and shape, color, and surface characteristics

Bilaterally equal or nearly equal, round or oval; wide variation of pigmentation, from light pink to dark brown; smooth with Montgomery's tubercles

DEVIATIONS: Grossly unequal; recent change in color; masses, lesions

Continued

Step	Normal/Individual Variations/Deviations
Nipples for size and shape, direction, color, and discharge	Bilaterally equal or nearly equal; slight flattening or retraction, easily everted with gentle pressure and no palpable mass; long-standing history of unilateral or bilateral inversion
	Pointing in equal direction; uniform color
	No discharge (NOTE: Some medications, such as tricyclic antidepressants, may cause a milky discharge.)
	DEVIATIONS: Grossly unequal; fixed inversion or retraction; deviation of nipple axis; redness, recent pigment changes; purulent, serous, or bloody discharge; crusting around nipple

Figures shown on pp. 183-186 from Malasanos L et al: *Health assessment,* ed 4, St Louis, 1990, Mosby.

Step	Normal/Individual Variations/Deviations
Reinspect above listed items in the following positions: Seated with arms extended overhead	As described above DEVIATIONS: Asymmetry, bulging, fixation, dimpling

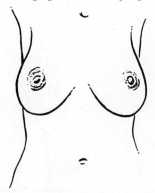

Seated and leaning forward from waist (support client by the hands)	

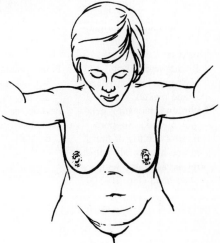

Continued

Step	Normal/Individual Variations/Deviations

Seated with hands on hips

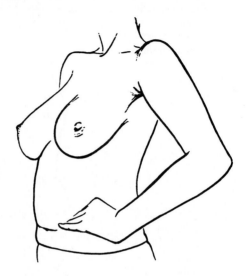

With client sitting upright, arms at sides or in lap, palpate

  Breasts and tail of Spence for consistency and masses

  Fine, granular consistency without masses; nontender; atrophy of tail of Spence

Technique (palpating pendlous breasts): Support inferior portion of breast in one hand while palpating breast tissue with other hand (Fig. 10-3).

DEVIATIONS: Unilateral mass, pain or tenderness, erythema

Step	Normal/Individual Variations/Deviations
(NOTE: If mass[es] identified, characterize by location, size, shape, consistency, discreteness, mobility, tenderness, erythema, and dimpling [see box, p. 188].)	

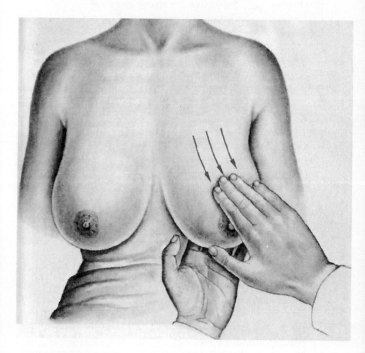

Fig. 10-3
Palpating large breasts. (From Seidel HM et al: *Mosby's guide to physical examination,* ed 3, St Louis, 1995, Mosby.)

Continued

Description of Breast Masses

Location:	By quadrant, or clock hour, with distance from the nipple
Size:	All dimensions, in centimeters
Shape:	Round or discoid, regular or irregular
Consistency:	Soft, firm, or hard
Discreteness:	Borders well or poorly defined
Mobility:	Movable in what direction(s) or fixed, with reference to skin and underlying tissue
Tenderness:	Subjective description or rating
Erythema:	Degree of redness
Dimpling:	Presence or absence; if present, describe location as noted above

Step	Normal/Individual Variations/Deviations
Lymph nodes	Nonpalpable
Technique: Relax muscles by slightly abducting and supporting the arm on side to be examined. Compress tissue between finger pads and chest wall using a firm, rolling motion. Palpate the following areas:	DEVIATION: Palpable
Deep axillary hollow	
Edge of pectoralis major along anterior axillary line	
Edge of latissimus dorsi along posterior axillary line	
Upper surface of humerus	
Subclavicular and supra-clavicular nodes	

Figures shown on pp. 183-186 from Malasanos L et al: *Health assessment,* ed 4, St Louis, 1990, Mosby.

Step	Normal/Individual Variations/Deviations
If nodes palpated, characterize as noted above for masses	
With client lying down, arm of breast to be examined placed behind head, and small pillow or folded towel under that shoulder to evenly displace breast tissue over chest wall (Fig. 10-4), palpate	

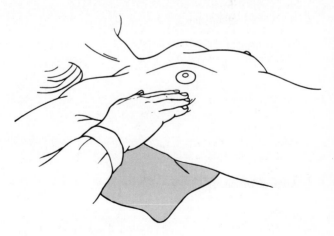

Fig. 10-4
Palpation of the breasts.

Continued

Step	Normal/Individual Variations/Deviations
Breasts and tail of Spence for consistency and masses	As described above DEVIATIONS: As described above
Technique: Consider the breast as a group of concentric circles with the nipple at the center. Starting at the outermost circle, palpate along the circumferences of each circle until the entire breast is examined (Fig. 10-5). Compress breast tissue between finger pads and chest wall, using a circular motion. Try not to lift palpating fingers off of the breast while moving from one area to the next. Perform a complete, light palpation, then proceed to deep palpation.	

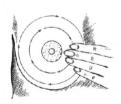

Fig. 10-5
Breast palpation technique, lying position. (From Phipps WJ et al: *Medical-surgical nursing*, ed 5, St Louis, 1995, Mosby.)

Step	Normal/Individual Variations/Deviations
Nipple for discharge and masses **Technique:** Gently compress the nipple with thumb and index finger in an attempt to express discharge. Use same technique to palpate for small masses.	As described above DEVIATIONS: As described above
Lymph nodes **Technique:** As described above.	As described above DEVIATIONS: As described above

Sample Documentation—Breast Mass

Health History

Mrs. D., 79, does not perform BSE and has never had a screening mammogram. Denies family history of breast cancer, breast discomfort, swelling/lumps, or nipple discharge. Onset of menarche age 14, menopause age 51. G_2 P_2 A_0. No history of hormone use or gynecologic surgery.

Physical Examination

Breasts large, pendulous, flabby; hanging low on chest wall; right slightly larger than left; slightly granular consistency with diffuse tenderness bilaterally; 1 cm × 1.5 cm × 1 cm round, soft, movable, well-delineated, tender mass palpated in RLQ at 4 o'clock, approximately 2 cm from nipple. Left nipple everted, right inverted (lifetime history); no discharge. Areolae equal and round, light brown. No lymphadenopathy.

Client Teaching

Self Breast Exam

1. The incidence of breast cancer increases with age. Just because your breasts atrophy with age does not mean you are risk-free for developing breast cancer. The atrophy of the glandular tissue in women over 65 years decreases the amount of palpable normal tissue in the breast, but malignancy can still develop.

2. Discuss the use of mammography as a screening tool with your health care practitioner at your next regularly scheduled health examination. Your health care practitioner will recommend the frequency with which you should have a screening mammogram.

3. Examine your breasts monthly, on the same day of the month. Pick a date that is easy to remember.

4. Begin by examining breasts while bathing or showering. Wet, soapy hands glide more easily over tissue.

5. Imagine your breast as the face of a clock. Start at 12 o'clock with your left fingertips at the top outermost portion of your right breast and begin palpating in a small, circular motion. Proceeding in a clockwise direction, move your fingertips to 1 o'clock and repeat. Keep moving around the clock, making smaller circles until reaching the nipple. Repeat procedure on left breast, using your right hand.

6. After bathing or showering, examine your breasts in front of a mirror, with your arms at your sides, with your hands on your hips with muscles flexed, with your arms over your head, and leaning over at the waist. Look for any swelling, dimpling of the skin, changes in the contour of the breasts, or changes in the nipples.

7. Next, examine your breasts lying down. To examine your right breast place a small pillow under your right shoulder, your right hand behind your head. Use the same procedure outlined in Number 5. Gently squeeze the nipple and observe for any discharge.

8. Report any changes to your health care practitioner immediately.

References

Malasanos L et al: *Health assessment,* ed 4, St Louis, 1990, Mosby.

Phipps WJ et al: *Medical-surgical nursing,* ed 5, St Louis, 1995, Mosby.

Seidel HM et al: *Mosby's guide to physical examination,* ed 3, St Louis, 1995, Mosby.

Thompson JM: *Clinical outlines for health assessment,* St Louis, 1997, Mosby.

Assessment of the Thorax and Lungs

11

Respiratory abnormalities and respiratory signs and symptoms occur more frequently in the older adult population because of multiple structural and functional changes in the thorax and lungs. Although age-related impairments occur in the respiratory system, adequate gaseous exchange can be maintained sufficiently in the absence of underlying pulmonary disease.

The sequence of assessment techniques is inspection, palpation, percussion, and auscultation. Refer to Chapter 3 for a detailed discussion of percussion and auscultation techniques. Equipment needs include a flexible pocket ruler, marking pen, and stethoscope with diaphragm and bell.

Surface landmarks of the thorax aid the examiner in describing the exact location of internal, underlying structures and findings. The examiner should become familiar with these landmarks to enhance the written description of assessment findings (see the box on pp. 195-196 and Fig. 11-1).

Anatomy and Physiology

The thorax, a semirigid cage surrounding the heart and lungs, is constructed of bone, cartilage, and muscle. The bony portions consist of 12 thoracic vertebrae, 12 paired ribs, and the sternum. The ribs are connected to the thoracic vertebrae posteriorly and to the sternum anteriorly. The body of the sternum attaches to the costal cartilages of the second through the tenth ribs. The costal cartilages of the eighth, ninth, and tenth ribs fuse to form the costal margin. Ribs eleven and twelve are floating ribs: their costal cartilages do not connect to any structures anteriorly.

The primary thoracic muscles are the diaphragm and intercostal muscles. The thoracic cage moves continuously with inspiration and expiration. During inspiration the diaphragm descends and flattens, thus lowering the abdominal contents and increasing intrathoracic space. The external intercostal muscles contract during inspiration, which elevates the anterior end of each rib, thus increasing the anteroposterior diameter of the chest. The internal intercostal muscles contract during expiration and pull the ribs down and in.

The shape of the thorax is essentially elliptical; its diameter is wider at the base than at the apex. The anteroposterior (AP) diam-

Anatomic and Thoracic Landmarks

The following anatomic markers on the chest are used to describe findings:
1. The nipples.
2. The manubriosternal junction (angle of Louis): a visible and palpable angulation of the sternum and the point at which the second rib articulates with the sternum. You can count the ribs and intercostal spaces from this point. The number of each intercostal space corresponds to that of the rib immediately above it.
3. The suprasternal notch: a depression, easily palpable and most often visible at the base of the ventral aspect of the neck, just superior to the manubriosternal junction.
4. Costal angle: the angle formed by the blending together of the costal margins at the sternum. It is usually no more than 90 degrees, with the ribs inserted at approximately 45-degree angles.
5. Vertebra prominens: the spinous process of C7. It can be more readily seen and felt when the patient's head is bent forward. If two prominences are felt, the upper is that of the spinous process of C7 and the lower is that of T1. It is difficult to use this as a guide for counting ribs posteriorly because the spinous processes from T4 down project obliquely, thus overlying the rib *below* the number of its vertebra.
6. The clavicles.

Continued

Anatomic and Thoracic Landmarks—cont'd

In conjunction with the anatomic landmarks of the chest, the following imaginary lines on the surface will help localize the findings on physical examination (Fig. 11-1):

1. Midsternal line: runs vertically down the midline of the sternum.
2. Right and left midclavicular lines: run parallel to the midsternal line, beginning at midclavicle; the inferior borders of the lungs generally cross the sixth rib at the midclavicular line.
3. Right and left anterior axillary lines: run parallel to the midsternal line, beginning at the anterior axillary folds.
4. Right and left midaxillary lines: run parallel to the midsternal line, beginning at the midaxilla.
5. Right and left posterior axillary lines: run parallel to the midsternal line, beginning at the posterior axillary folds.
6. Midspinal line: runs vertically down the spinal processes.
7. Right and left scapular lines: run parallel to the midspinal line, through the inferior angle of the scapula, when the patient is erect.

Modified from Seidel HM et al: *Mosby's guide to physical examination,* ed 3, St Louis, 1995, Mosby.

eter of the thorax is less than the transverse diameter by an approximate ratio of between 1:2 and 5:7.

The thoracic cavity is divided into the right and left pleural cavities and the mediastinum (Fig. 11-2). The pleural cavities are lined by the visceral pleura, or lung layer, and the parietal pleura, or wall layer; the pleural cavity is the space between these pleural layers. A small amount of fluid within each of the pleural cavities acts as a lubricant to allow the lungs to slide along the chest wall. The lungs are separated from one another by the mediastinum. The mediastinum is the region posterior to the body of the sternum, and it contains the heart, great vessels, aortic arch, and thoracic aorta; many arteries, veins, and nerves; the esophagus; the trachea; and the two main bronchi.

The lungs are large, spongy, paired but asymmetric organs that conform to the thoracic cavity. The right lung has three lobes; the

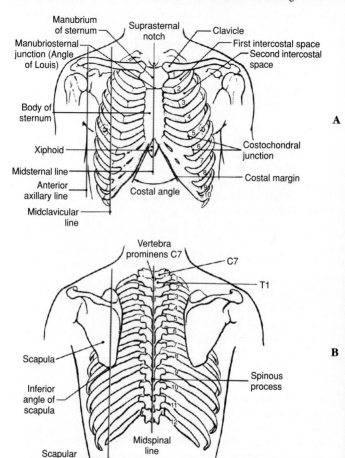

Fig. 11-1
Topographic landmarks. **A,** Anterior thorax. **B,** Posterior thorax. (From Malasanos L et al: *Health assessment,* ed 4, St Louis, 1990, Mosby.)   *Continued*

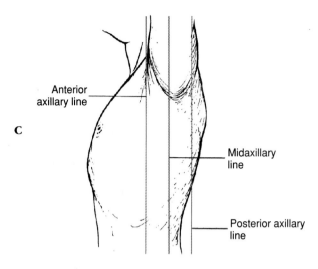

Anterior
axillary line

C

Midaxillary
line

Posterior axillary
line

Fig. 11-1, cont'd
C, Lateral thorax. (From Malasanos L et al: *Health assessment,* ed 4,
St Louis, 1990, Mosby.)

left, two. The lungs lie against the rib cage anteriorly and posteriorly and extend from the diaphragm to just above the clavicles. All structures of the respiratory system beyond the bronchi are contained within the lungs.

Air reaches and leaves the lung via the tracheobronchial tree, which consists of the trachea (Chapter 7), right and left main bronchi, bronchioles, and alveoli. The trachea bifurcates into the right and left bronchi. The right bronchus is shorter, wider, and more vertical than the left; it divides into three branches that supply the three lobes of the right lung. The left bronchus divides into two branches that supply the two lobes of the left lung. The bronchi continue to subdivide until they become the microscopic alveoli, where gaseous exchange between the external environment and the blood occurs. Adult lungs contain as many as 300 million alveoli.

Respiration

The purpose of respiration is to exchange oxygen and carbon dioxide between the external environment and the blood. The regula-

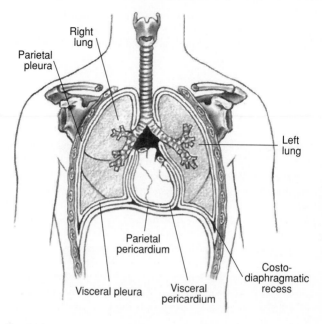

Fig. 11-2
Related structures of the chest cavity, anterior view. (From Thompson JM et al: *Mosby's clinical nursing,* ed 4, St Louis, 1997, Mosby.)

tion of the respiratory cycle is highly complex. The rhythmicity of breathing is controlled by neurons in the reticular formation of the medulla oblongata. The firing of certain neurons produces inspiration, whereas that of other neurons produces expiration. This cycle of activity is influenced by two centers in the pons. Central chemoreceptors located in the medulla oblongata that respond to changes in pH in the cerebrospinal fluid also affect respiration. Peripheral chemoreceptors, including the aortic bodies located in the aortic arch and the carotid bodies, also respond to changes in arterial oxygen and carbon dioxide levels. These peripheral chemoreceptors affect breathing by stimulating the respiratory centers to initiate reflexive ventilation.

The lungs also contain various types of receptors that influence the brainstem respiratory control centers via sensory fibers in the vagus nerve. For example, irritant receptors stimulate reflex constriction of bronchioles in response to irritation from noxious agents. Also, stretch receptors activated by inspiration inhibit the respiratory control centers, making further inspiration increasingly difficult. Expiration then begins, and the lungs recoil.

Aging causes many structural and functional changes of both the thorax and lungs. Alveoli become less elastic and more fibrous and contain fewer functional capillaries, so the body's exertional capacity decreases because the lungs' diffusion capacity for oxygen cannot meet the body's demands. Loss of lung resiliency, which normally holds the thorax in a slightly contracted position, coupled with the loss of skeletal muscle strength in the thorax and diaphragm, results in the characteristic barrel chest. Decalcification of ribs and increased calcification of the costal cartilages also occur. Because of the more rigid thoracic wall and weaker muscles of respiration, the ability to cough effectively is decreased. Kyphosis, an increase in thoracic spine curvature caused by wedging of the thoracic vertebrae and thinning of the intervertebral disks, coupled with a loss of lumbar curvature, is often accompanied by an increased AP diameter. Drier mucous membranes impede removal of secretions and create greater risk of respiratory infection.

Assessment of the Thorax and Lungs

Equipment needed:
    Flexible pocket ruler
    Marking pen
    Stethoscope

Step	Normal/Individual Variations/Deviations
With client sitting on edge of examination table, disrobed to waist (provide drape for female during posterior examination), inspect	
Chest shape and symmetry	Slightly convex with no sternal depression
	Downward and equal slope of ribs

Step	Normal/Individual Variations/Deviations
	Costal angle slightly less than 90 degrees
	Symmetric landmarks
	Marked bony prominences, decreased subcutaneous fat
	1:2 to 5:7 ratio, or may have increased AP diameter (kyphosis)
	DEVIATIONS: Retraction, localized bulges, sternal depressions; horizontal ribs; costal angle greater than 90 degrees; asymmetric landmarks; barrel chest
Skin characteristics	Even color consistent with other body parts
	DEVIATIONS: Pallor, cyanosis, spider nevi
Respiratory rate and rhythm	12 to 20 respirations per minute, unlabored
	Chest expansion bilaterally symmetric; duration of inspiration slightly longer than that of expiration
	Breathes easily and regularly without distress
	DEVIATIONS: Tachypnea, hyperpnea, bradypnea; chest asymmetry; expiration prolonged and labored; may alternate with periods of shallow breathing; labored, irregular, painful breathing; use of accessory muscles in the neck (sternocleidomastoid, scalenus, and trapezius), and supraclavicular retraction

Continued

Step	Normal/Individual Variations/Deviations
Palpate	
Tracheal alignment	Trachea in midline
Technique: Place index finger in suprasternal notch and gently move it side to side in space bordered by upper edge of clavicle, inner aspect of sternocleidomastoid muscle and trachea.	DEVIATIONS: Lateral deviations of trachea
General chest wall characteristics	Skin warm and smooth No tenderness, bulges, depressions, crepitus, vibration, or abnormal movement DEVIATIONS: Skin cold or hot, excessively dry or moist; tenderness, masses, crepitus, or coarse grating vibration
Thoracic expansion	Symmetric movement of thumbs
Technique: Place your thumbs along spinal processes at level of tenth rib, palms along posterolateral thorax. Instruct client to breathe normally, and observe movement of thumbs; next instruct client to breathe deeply, and observe again.	DEVIATIONS: Unequal movement of thumbs

Step	Normal/Individual Variations/Deviations
Tactile fremitus **Technique:** While systematically palpating thorax with ulnar aspect of one hand or ulnar aspect of closed fist, instruct client to say "one, two, three" or "ninety-nine." Compare one side to the other; do not test over bone.	Varies depending on intensity and pitch of voice. Bilaterally equal, mild vibration with greater intensity at anterior and posterior base of neck and along trachea and large bronchi DEVIATIONS: Increased vibration palpated (pneumonia, compressed lung, tumor); decreased or absent vibration palpated (pleural effusion or thickening, pneumothorax, bronchial obstruction, or emphysema)
Percuss posterior, lateral, and anterior chest wall **Technique:** (see Chapter 3 for review of percussion method) Instruct client to sit with head bent forward and arms folded in front to spread scapulae and expose more lung area for posterior percussion. Next have client sit straight while raising arms overhead for lateral and anterior chest percussion (see Fig. 11-3 for sequence for systematic percussion).	Resonance throughout lung fields; may hear hyperresonance secondary to increased lung distensibility (refer to physician for further evaluation) DEVIATIONS: Dullness or extreme hyperresonance

Continued

Step	Normal/Individual Variations/Deviations
Diaphragmatic excursion **Technique:** Instruct client to breathe two normal, full respirations, then take a third deep breath and hold it. Starting at the apex of the right scapula, quickly percuss down posterior chest along scapular line until lower edge of lung is identified (sound will change from resonance to dullness). Identify that point with marking pen, and instruct client to breathe. Allowing sufficient time for recovery, instruct client to exhale completely, then hold breath. Again, percuss up from the marked point until that tone changes and mark that point (sound will change from dullness to resonance). Repeat procedure on left side. Measure and record distance from the upper to the lower point on each side.	Bilateral excursion ranging from 3 to 5 cm, slightly higher on the left DEVIATIONS: Asymmetric response or extremely limited excursion overall

Step	Normal/Individual Variations/Deviations
Auscultate posterior, lateral, and anterior chest wall **Technique:** Instruct client to sit upright with head bent forward and arms folded in front, then to breathe slowly and deeply through the mouth (demonstrate if necessary). Caution client to stop if discomfort or lightheadedness occurs. Place diaphragm of stethoscope firmly on skin, and listen to the inspiratory and expiratory phases at each position (Fig. 11-3). Compare sounds from side to side while moving from apex to base.	Vesicular breath sounds over most of posterior lung fields Bronchovesicular breath sounds in the areas of the major bronchi, but especially over upper right posterior lung field (Table 11-1) DEVIATIONS: Bronchovesicular or bronchial breath sounds over peripheral lung fields; adventitious sounds (see Table 11-2 on pp. 208-209)
Next have client sit upright with arms overhead for lateral chest auscultation.	Vesicular breath sounds (Table 11-1) DEVIATIONS: Bronchovesicular breath sounds; no breath sounds
Finally, have client sit upright with shoulder thrust back for anterior chest auscultation.	Vesicular breath sounds over peripheral lung fields, bronchial breath sounds over trachea, and bronchovesicular breath sounds over main bronchi (Table 11-1) DEVIATIONS: Bronchovesicular and bronchial breath sounds over peripheral lung fields; adventitious sounds (see Table 11-2 on pp. 208-209)

Continued

Step	Normal/Individual Variations/Deviations
Assess resonance if abnormality detected on palpation of tactile fremitus:	
Whispered pectoriloquy	Muffled, nondistinct sound that is loudest medially, less intense at periphery of lung
Technique: While listening with stethoscope (using sequence for systematic auscultation), instruct client to whisper "ninety-nine" or "one, two, three."	DEVIATIONS: Clarity of sound; present in any condition that causes lung consolidation
Egophony	Muffled "eee" sound
Technique: While listening, instruct client to say "eee."	DEVIATIONS: "ay" sound
Bronchophony	Muffled sound
Technique: While listening, instruct client to say "ninety-nine" or "one, two, three."	DEVIATIONS: Clarity of sound

Table 11-1   Characteristics of normal breath sounds

Sound	Characteristics
Vesicular	Heard over most of lung fields; low pitch; soft and short expirations
Bronchovesicular	Heard over main bronchus area and over upper right posterior lung field; medium pitch; expiration equals inspiration
Bronchial	Heard only over trachea; high pitch; loud and long expirations

From Thompson JM et al: *Mosby's clinical nursing,* ed 3, St Louis, 1993, Mosby.

Sample Documentation—Pneumonia

Health History

Daughter of Mrs. R., 81, notes a decrease in Mrs. R.'s usual activity level and attention span for past 3 days and feels she is becoming more lethargic. Also having difficulty sleeping at night because of persistent dry cough; earlier today noted cough becoming productive of purulent green sputum. No fever. Appetite decreased.

Physical Examination

Thin, pale, apathetic-appearing female. Responds sluggishly to questions. Oriented to place and person. BP 118/60, P 92/min, R 32/minute and shallow, T 98.4° F. Trachea in midline. Marked kyphosis. Thoracic expansion symmetric. Increased tactile fremitus LLL with increased percussed dullness. Diaphragmatic excursion 2 cm L, 4 cm R. Diminished breath sounds LLL posteriorly with inspiratory coarse crackles; increased egophony and bronchophony. R posterior lung fields CTA without adventitious sounds, and with resonant percussion tones.

Table 11-2 Adventitious breath sounds

Sound/Description	Clinical Significance	Common Conditions	Nursing Implications
Wheeze—continuous (>250 ms) high-pitched (sibilant) or low-pitched (sonorous) sound caused when the airway narrows to the point at which opposite walls touch; sibilant wheezes originate is small bronchioles and often occur in late expiration; sonorous wheezes originate in larger bronchi and usually heard in early expiration	Caused by bronchospasm, the presence of mucus, or edema of the airway; can be associated with airway plugging, tumor, or foreign body; frequently clears with coughing	Asthma; acute bronchitis; emphysema; cor pulmonale; pneumonia	Report assessment findings; assess for shortness of breath; administer bronchodilators; provide chest physiotherapy/postural drainage (CPT/PD); provide pulmonary hygiene measures of suctioning, coughing, and deep breathing

Crackle—discontinuous sound (20 ms); series of brief, explosive sounds; dry quality; may be heard more on inspiration; fine crackles are high-pitched, occur late in inspiration, and reflect air passing through moisture in bronchioles and alveoli; medium-pitched crackles occur in midinspiration-and reflect air passing through moisture in small bronchi; coarse crackles are low-pitched, occur early in inspiration, and reflect air passing through moisture in larger bronchi	Presence of mucus, pus, or fluid in airway (NOTE: Crackles caused by cardiac failure are gravity dependent and will move throughout the thorax relative to patient positioning; they are not cleared by cough.)	Atelectasis; bronchiectasis; emphysema; pneumonia; pulmonary fibrosis; pulmonary edema; congestive heart failure; cor pulmonale; tumor	Report assessment findings; determine whether the crackles result from pulmonary or cardiac causes
Pleural friction rub—cracking, grating sound heard during inspiration or expiration	Indicates area of pleural inflammation or roughened pleural surfaces; coughing has no effect	Pleural effusion; pneumonia	Report findings to physician

Modified from Wellitz PB: *Pocket guide to respiratory care*, St Louis, 1991, Mosby.

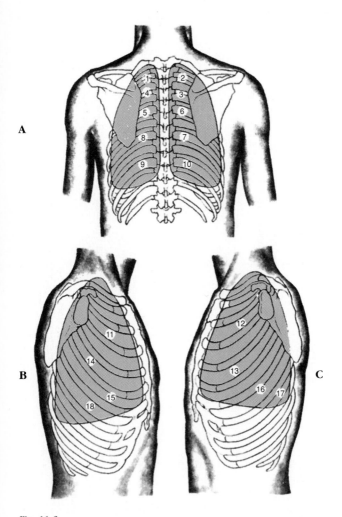

Fig. 11-3
Sequence for percussion and auscultation of the chest. (From Talbot L, Meyers-Marquardt M: *Pocket guide to critical care assessment,* ed 3, St Louis, 1997, Mosby.)   *Continued*

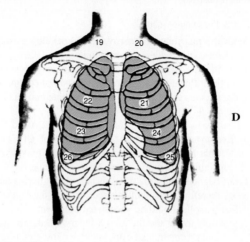

Fig. 11-3, cont'd
Sequence for percussion and auscultation of the chest. (From Talbot L, Meyers-Marquardt M: *Pocket guide to critical care assessment,* ed 3, St Louis, 1997, Mosby.)

Client Teaching

Influenza Prevention

1. Influenza or the "flu" can be a serious, life-threatening condition in older persons and in those with chronic illness. Consequently, it is important for older persons to protect themselves from this disease by getting yearly immunization.

2. The flu is a viral infection of the respiratory tract that is highly contagious. Sometimes it is difficult to tell the difference between a simple cold and the flu. Usually a fever does not accompany a cold, and a stuffy nose occurs more often with a cold than with the flu. A cold, although an uncomfortable nuisance, is associated with symptoms that are usually much milder and do not last as long as the symptoms of the flu.

Continued

Client Teaching

Influenza Prevention—cont'd

3. With the flu, you will feel weak and develop a cough, headache, and sudden rise in temperature. Other symptoms include widespread aching, chills, and occasional vomiting. Pneumonia is a common complication, and older persons are at risk for developing pneumonia along with the flu.

4. There are two major types of influenza: Type A and Type B. Every year the Centers for Disease Control (CDC) projects what types of influenza will likely be prevalent in the upcoming year, and production of vaccine for those types begins. The virus types usually differ from year to year: therefore a flu shot is effective only for 1 year.

5. Older persons should be vaccinated in the early fall. It is impossible to get the flu from a flu shot. Side effects to the vaccine sometimes occur, such as a low-grade fever and redness/tenderness at the injection site, both of which can be relieved by aspirin or acetaminophen. Influenza vaccine should never be given to those who are allergic to eggs, since the vaccine is made in egg products.

6. If you get the flu, call your health care practitioner immediately. An antiviral drug, amantidine, may be prescribed. Aspirin and acetaminophen may be recommended for the aches, pains, and fever. Drink plenty of fluids and get plenty of rest; stay in bed for 1 to 2 days after the fever has subsided. Amantidine is used as a preventative and may be warranted if you do not have the flu but have been exposed to someone who does have the flu.

Compiled from *What to do about flu,* Age Page, National Institute on Aging, Bethesda, Md, 1991, US Department of Health and Human Services, Public Health Service, National Institutes of Health.

References

Malasanos L et al: *Health assessment,* ed 4, St Louis, 1990, Mosby.

Seidel HM et al: *Mosby's guide to physical examination,* ed 3, St Louis, 1995, Mosby.

Talbot L, Meyers-Marquardt M: *Pocket guide to critical care assessment,* ed 3, St Louis, 1997, Mosby.

Thompson JM et al: *Mosby's clinical nursing,* ed 4, St Louis, 1997, Mosby.

Weilitz PB: *Pocket guide to respiratory care,* St Louis, 1991, Mosby.

What to do about flu, Age Page, National Institute on Aging, Bethesda, Md, 1991. US Department of Health and Human Services, Public Health Service, National Institutes of Health.

Assessment of the Heart and Vascular System

12

The main components of the cardiovascular system are the heart and vasculature. Assessment of the vascular system is discussed here; however, this assessment is usually integrated throughout the physical examination.

Although there is a higher incidence of cardiovascular disease in older adults, the nurse should not assume that all older persons have disease or impairment. Careful symptom analysis is of prime importance when assessing the heart. The techniques of inspection, palpation, percussion, and auscultation are used. Equipment needs include a centimeter ruler, penlight, stethoscope with bell and diaphragm, and sphygmomanometer.

Anatomy and Physiology

The Heart

Several anterior chest wall landmarks are important in examination of the heart and description of findings (Fig. 12-1). The heart lies in the thoracic cavity within the mediastinum. In general, it is behind the sternum, but the exact position varies, depending on individual body build, chest configuration, and diaphragm level. The two atria make up the base of the heart, which lies at the top behind the upper portion of the sternum. The two ventricles comprise the apex of the heart, which is positioned downward and toward the left. The aorta, pulmonary arteries, and great veins are located around the base of the heart (Fig. 12-1).

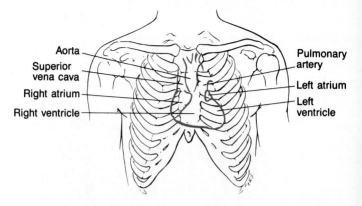

Fig. 12-1
Chest wall landmarks. (Redrawn from Malasanos L et al: *Health assessment,* ed 4, St Louis, 1990, Mosby.)

The heart is encased in a strong, double-walled fibrous sac called the pericardium. The outer layer of the pericardium is firmly attached within the thorax to the esophagus, aorta, pleura, sternum, and diaphragm. A small amount of serous fluid between the two layers of pericardium reduces the friction of the constantly moving heart muscle.

The heart itself is composed of three layers. The epicardium is a thin, smooth lining that covers the outside of the myocardium and interfaces with the inner layer of the pericardium. The myocardium is the thick, muscular middle layer. The endocardium is a thin, delicate membrane that lines the heart chambers and the surfaces of the heart valves.

Blood flow through the four chambers of the heart is regulated by two sets of valves: the atrioventricular (AV) valves, which are between the chambers on each side, and the semilunar valves, which are at the points where blood leaves the heart (Fig. 12-2). The valves maintain the forward flow of blood at all times by responding to pressure gradients, passively opening and closing. The AV valves, located between the atria and ventricles, include the tricuspid and mitral valves. The tricuspid valve is composed of three thin, translucent leaflets, and it separates the right atrium from the right ventricle. The mitral valve is composed of two thicker, less translucent leaflets, and it separates the left atrium from the left

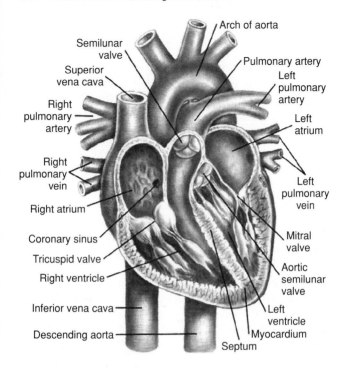

Fig. 12-2
Frontal schematic section of the heart. (From Thompson JM et al: *Mosby's clinical nursing,* ed 4, St Louis, 1997, Mosby.)

ventricle. When atrial pressure is higher than ventricular pressure, the atria contract and the AV valves open, allowing blood to fill the ventricles. When ventricular pressure is higher than atrial pressure, the AV valves close, preventing blood from flowing back up into the atria. The semilunar valves are the pulmonic and aortic valves. The pulmonic valve separates the right ventricle from the pulmonary artery; the aortic valve separates the left ventricle from the aorta. When ventricular pressure is higher than atrial pressure, the ventricles contract and the semilunar valves open, allowing blood to flow into the pulmonary artery and aorta. When ventricular pressure is lower than atrial pressure, the ventricles relax and fill with blood. This decreased pressure causes the semilunar valves to close.

Attached to the AV valve leaflets are the papillary muscles and chordae tendineae. Each leaflet is held in position by the chordae

Timing and duration*	
Early systolic	Begins with S_1, decrescendo, ends well before S_2
Midsystolic (ejection)	Begins after S_1, ends before S_2; crescendo-decrescendo quality sometimes difficult to discern
Late systolic	Begins mid to late systole, crescendo, ends at S_2; often introduced by mid- to late-systolic clicks
Early diastolic	Begins with S_2
Middiastolic	Begins at clear interval after S_2
Late diastolic (presystolic)	Begins immediately before S_1
Holosystolic (pansystolic)	Begins with S_1, occupies all of systole, ends at S_2
Holodiastolic (pandiastolic)	Begins with S_2, occupies all of diastole, ends at S_1
Continuous	Starts in systole, continues without interruption through S_2 into all or part of diastole; does not necessarily persist throughout entire cardiac cycle

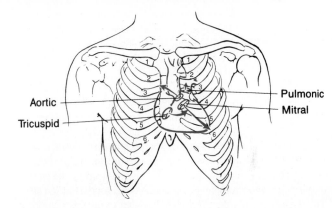

Fig. 12-3

Transmission of closure sounds from the heart valves to the surface of the chest. (From Malasanos L et al: *Health assessment,* ed 4, St Louis, 1990, Mosby.)

tendineae, which are strong, tendinous cords of fibrous tissue secured to the ventricular wall by the cone-shaped papillary muscles. These structures keep the valves from everting when the ventricles contract.

Heart sounds are produced principally by valve closure, but the areas on the chest wall where closure is best heard are not located directly over the valves (Fig. 12-3). The areas where valve closure can best be auscultated are the following:

Aortic valve: second right intercostal space at the sternal border

Pulmonic valve: second left intercostal space at the sternal border

Tricuspid valve: fourth left intercostal space at the lower left sternal border

Mitral valve: fifth left intercostal space at the midclavicular line

The great vessels lying at the base of the heart circulate blood through the heart and lungs in a consistent rhythmic fashion. The great vessels include the superior and inferior vena cava, the pulmonary artery and veins, and the aorta. Blood enters the right atrium from the systemic circulation via the superior and inferior vena cava. It flows from the right atrium, through the tricuspid valve, and into the right ventricle. Blood is then pumped through the pulmonic valve into the pulmonary artery, which bifurcates into the right and left branches, which in turn lead to the lungs.

Oxygenated blood leaves the lungs via the right and left pulmonary veins. The blood passes into the left atrium, through the mitral valve, and into the left ventricle. The left ventricle then pumps blood to the body through the aortic valve and aorta (Fig. 12-4).

Cardiac Cycle

The classic heart sounds are discrete, brief auditory vibrations of varying intensity, frequency, quality, and duration: they are related to events in the cardiac cycle. The first heart sound (S_1) corresponds to the onset of ventricular systole, when ventricular contraction increases the pressure in the ventricles and forces the AV valves closed. This characteristic "lubb" sound is produced by the closure of the mitral and tricuspid valves and is heard loudest at the apex. The pressure within the ventricles continues to increase until it is greater than that in the aorta and pulmonary artery, at which point the aortic and pulmonic valves open, ejecting blood into the arteries. This is the force known as *afterload*. The second heart sound (S_2) corresponds to the onset of diastole and is caused by the closure

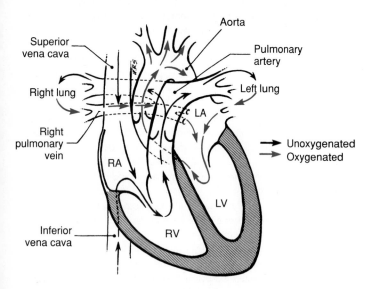

Fig. 12-4
Route of blood flow through the chambers of the heart and the great vessels. (From Malasanos L et al: *Health assessment*, ed 4, St Louis, 1990, Mosby.)

of the aortic and pulmonic valves. Th
est at the base. During diastole, the
challenged to relax and fill; the force
place is termed *preload*. A longer |
S_1 than between S_1 and S_2. These ev
heart, but only slightly later on the ri
and fourth heart sounds of low freque
and may be indicative of serious hea

Other Heart Sounds

S_3 occurs in rapid ventricular diasto
soon after S_2. The sound is accentuate
position; it is heard best at the apex
scope. An S_3 may signify early conge
person. The S_4 sound occurs in late c
sult of forceful atrial contraction to er
a low-frequency sound, is heard best
be heard in any location. It results fro
ing secondary to a change in ventricu
increase; thus in older adults, it may l
sive cardiovascular disease, coronary
sis, or severe anemia. When S_3 and S
with severe myocardial disease and ta
a summation gallop.

Heart murmurs, abnormal sounds d
produced by vibration within the hear
sels. Frequently the cause is an abno
valve; therefore the murmur is best he
murs are produced by the following thr
bination: (1) increased rate of blood flo
forward blood flow through irregular o
a dilated blood vessel or chamber, and
flow through an incompetent valve, sep
arteriosus. Refer to Table 12-1, pp. 220-
characteristics of heart murmurs.

Conduction System

An electrical conduction system coordi
diac events. An electrical impulse origin
sinoatrial (SA) node, located in the right
els through both atria to the AV node, wl
septum. The impulse moves on through

Table 12-1   Characterization of heart murmurs

Pitch	High, medium, low	Depends on pressure and rate of blood flow; low pitch is heard best with the bell
Intensity†	Grade I	Barely audible in quiet room
	Grade II	Quiet but clearly audible
	Grade III	Moderately loud
	Grade IV	Loud, associated with thrill
	Grade V	Very loud, thrill easily palpable
	Grade VI	Very loud, audible with stethoscope not in contact with chest, thrill palpable and visible
Pattern	Crescendo	Increasing intensity caused by increased blood velocity
	Decrescendo	Decreasing intensity caused by decreased blood velocity
Quality	Harsh, raspy, machinelike, vibratory, musical, blowing	Quality depends on several factors, including degree of valve compromise, force of contractions, blood volume

*Systolic murmurs are best described according to time of onset and termination; diastolic murmurs are best classified according to time of onset only.

†Discrimination among the six grades is more difficult for the diastolic murmur than for the systolic.

Continued

Table 12-1 Characterization of heart murmurs—cont'd

	Classification	Description
Location	Anatomic landmarks (e.g., second left intercostal space on sternal border)	Area of greatest intensity, usually area to which valve sounds are normally transmitted
Radiation	Anatomic landmarks (e.g., to axilla)	Site farthest from location of greatest intensity at which sound is still heard; sound usually transmitted in direction of blood flow
Respiratory phase variations	Intensity, quality, and timing variable	Venous return increases on inspiration and decreases on expiration

From Seidel HM et al: *Mosby's guide to physical examination*, ed 3, St Louis, 1995, Mosby.

branches into the ventricular myocardium, stimulating ventricular contraction. An electrocardiogram (ECG) is a graphic recording of this electrical activity (Fig. 12-5). The P wave represents electrical invasion of the atria, or atrial depolarization. The P-R interval is the time taken for the impulse to pass from the SA node to the ventricle. The QRS complex represents the spread of the impulse through the ventricles, or ventricular depolarization. The S-T segment and T wave represent the return of the ventricular muscle to a resting state, or ventricular repolarization.

Peripheral Circulation

The peripheral circulation consists of the arterial and venous systems. Arteries are tougher, have greater tensile strength, and are less distensible than veins. The vasomotor center in the brain selectively constricts and dilates the arteries, which thus regulates blood flow to the appropriate tissue beds based on need. Veins are less sturdy and more passive than arteries. Because the blood pressure within them is low, veins have adaptations to keep venous return to the heart equal to cardiac output. The large-diameter lu-

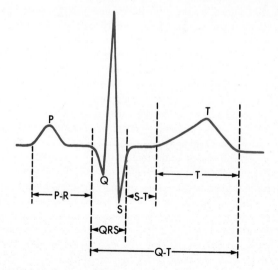

Fig. 12-5
Normal electrocardiographic waveform. (From Berne RM, Levy MN: *Physiology,* ed 3, St Louis, 1993, Mosby.)

mens of veins and the presence of valves are two such structural adaptations. Coupled with the massaging action of skeletal muscle activity, blood is kept flowing toward the heart.

Because the carotid arteries and jugular veins are the most accessible vessels that are close to the heart, examination of these vessels provides valuable information about heart function. Assessment of peripheral pulses (superficial temporal, brachial, radial, femoral, popliteal, dorsalis pedis, and posterior tibial) gives less information about left ventricular ejection or aortic valvular function than does assessment of the carotids. However, assessment of the rate, amplitude, rhythm, and symmetry of peripheral pulses gives an indication of cardiac function and peripheral tissue perfusion.

The heart of a normal older adult without hypertension or clinical disease remains the same size or becomes slightly smaller than it was in middle age. Overall, the heart rate slows, stroke volume decreases, and cardiac output is reduced by 30% to 40%. Occasional ectopic beats are common and may or may not indicate a pathologic condition.

Sclerosis and thickening of the valve leaflets occur particularly in the mitral and aortic valves. The endocardium thickens and scleroses; the myocardium becomes more rigid and slower in recovering its contractility and irritability. Consequently, sudden or prolonged stress and tachycardia are poorly tolerated. The heart rate elevation in response to stress is reduced, and an elevated heart rate takes longer to return to baseline. To compensate for the sluggish increase in heart rate, the stroke volume may increase. This increases cardiac output, which may result in elevated blood pressure.

The tunica media layer of the muscular and coronary arteries calcifies and loses elasticity. This calcification causes dilation and tortuosity of the aorta, aortic branches, and carotid arteries. Early, soft systolic murmurs may be heard as a result of these changes. The superficial vessels of the forehead, neck, and extremities also become tortuous and more prominent. Systolic blood pressure increases in response to the loss of elasticity in the peripheral vessels and subsequent increase in peripheral vascular resistance. The increasing lability of vasopressor action raises both systolic and diastolic pressures.

According to the *Fifth Report of the Joint National Committee on Detection, Evaluation, and Treatment of High Blood Pressure* (1993), the prevalence of isolated systolic hypertension (ISH), defined as systolic blood pressure (SBP) of 140 mm Hg or greater and diastolic blood pressure (DBP) less than 90 mm Hg, increases after age 60. A number of studies reported in the above publication have established the value of treating hypertension in older persons. The goal of therapy is to decrease the SBP to <160 mm Hg if the pressure is >180 mm Hg and to reduce blood pressure by 20 mm Hg for those with SBP between 160 and 179 mm Hg. If ISH is between 140 and 160 mm Hg, then life-style modifications or definitive therapy is indicated. The goals of therapy for DBP remain the same as those established for the general population (see the table below).

Vasomotor tone and baroreceptor sensitivity decrease. Vagal tone increases, which decreases heart rate. The myocardium is less sensitive to atropine and more sensitive to carotid sinus stimulation.

A decrease in hemoglobin is a frequent finding among older adults. Poor dietary intake, secondary to loneliness, structural alterations in the mouth and oropharynx, gastrointestinal system

Classification of blood pressure for adults age 18 years and older*

Category	Systolic (mm Hg)	Diastolic (mm Hg)
Normal†	<130	<85
High normal	130-139	85-89
Hypertension‡		
Stage 1 (mild)	140-159	90-99
Stage 2 (moderate)	160-179	100-109
Stage 3 (severe)	180-209	110-119
Stage 4 (very severe)	≥210	≥120

From National Institutes of Health, 1993.

*Not taking antihypertensive drugs and not acutely ill. When systolic and diastolic pressures fall into different categories, the higher category should be selected to classify the individual's blood pressure status. For instance, 160/92 mm Hg should be classified as stage 2, and 180/120 mm Hg should be classified as stage 4. Isolated systolic hypertension (ISH) is defined as SBP ≥140 mm Hg and DBP <90 mm Hg and staged appropriately (e.g., 170/85 mm Hg is defined as stage 2 ISH).

†Optimal blood pressure with respect to cardiovascular risk is SBP <120 mm Hg and DBP <80 mm Hg. However, unusually low readings should be evaluated for clinical significance.

‡Based on the average of two or more readings taken at each of two or more visits following an initial screening.

NOTE: In addition to classifying stages of hypertension based on average blood pressure levels, the clinician should specify presence or absence of target-organ disease and additional risk factors. For example, a patient with diabetes and a blood pressure of 142/94 mm Hg plus left ventricular hypertrophy should be classified as "stage 1 hypertension with target-organ disease (left ventricular hypertrophy) and with another major risk factor (diabetes)." This specificity is important for risk classification and management.

changes that affect absorption, and chronic disease may be contributing factors to anemia, which results in a decrease in the concentration of oxygen that can be transported by blood.

Electrocardiographic changes may occur as a result of cellular changes, fibrotic changes within the conduction system, and neurogenic changes. There is a slight prolongation of all intervals and a possible decreased voltage of all waves.

Assessment of the Heart and Vascular System

Equipment needed:
    Centimeter ruler
    Penlight
    Stethoscope
    Sphygmomanometer

Step	Normal/Individual Variations/Deviations
With client lying down, palpate superficial temporal, carotid, brachial, radial, femoral, popliteal, dorsalis pedis, and posterior tibial pulses for rate, rhythm, amplitude, contour, and symmetry (Table 12-2) **Technique** (carotid artery palpation): Place distal pads of first three fingers just under mandible, between trachea and sternocleidomastoid muscle, and instruct client to flex neck slightly and rotate toward side being examined. Never palpate both sides simultaneously, and avoid excess pressure. Document amplitude based on following scale: 0 = absent; 1^+ = diminished, weak, thready; 2^+ = normal; 3^+ = bounding.	60 to 90 beats/minute Regular rhythm or regularly irregular; prompt, smooth, and rounded upstroke; symmetric in all of the above responses DEVIATIONS: Less than 60 or more than 90 beats/minute; unpredictably irregular; bounding, diminishing, or absent upstroke; asymmetric in any one of these characteristics (see Table 12-3 for further descriptions of deviations)

Step	Normal/Individual Variations/Deviations
Measure blood pressure in both arms	90/60 to 139/89 mm Hg, or up to 159/89 mm Hg if stable over a period of time, if client is asymptomatic, and if client does not show evidence of end organ damage; 30 to 40 mm Hg pulse pressure; pressures in both arms the same or with variance no greater than 5 to 10 mm Hg

Continued

Table 12-2   Locations of palpable pulses

Pulse	Location
Superficial temporal	Anterior to the ear, over the temporal muscle, and into the forehead
Carotid	In the neck, just medial to and below angle of the jaw (do not palpate both sides simultaneously)
Brachial	Just medial to biceps tendon
Radial	Medial and ventral side of wrist (gentle pressure)
Femoral	Inferior and medial to inguinal ligament; if patient is obese, midway between anterior superior iliac spine and pubic tubercle (press harder here than in most areas)
Popliteal	Popliteal fossae (press firmly)
Dorsalis pedis	Medial side of dorsum of foot with foot slightly dorsiflexed (pulse may be hard to feel and may be absent even in some well persons)
Posterior tibial	Behind and slightly inferior to medial malleolus of ankle (pulse may be hard to feel and may not be palpable in some well persons)

Modified from Seidel HM et al: *Mosby's guide to physical examination,* ed 3, St Louis, 1995, Mosby.

Table 12-3 Arterial pulse abnormalities

Type	Description	Associated Disorders
Alternating pulse (pulsus alternans)	Regular rate; amplitude varies from beat to beat with weak and strong beats	Left ventricular failure
Bisferious pulse (pulsus bisferiens)	Two strong systolic peaks separated by a midsystolic dip	Aortic regurgitation alone or with stenosis
Bigeminal pulse (pulsus bigeminus)	Two beats in rapid succession followed by longer interval; easily confused with alternating pulse	Regularly occurring ventricular premature beats
Bounding pulse	Increased pulse pressure; contour may have rapid rise, brief peak, rapid fall	Atherosclerosis, aortic regurgitation, patent ductus arteriosus, fever, anemia, hyperthyroidism, anxiety, exercise
Bradycardia	Rate less than 60 bpm	Hypothermia, hypothyroidism, drug intoxication, impaired cardiac conduction, excellent physical conditioning

Labile pulse	Normal when patient is resting but faster when standing or sitting	Not necessarily associated with disease; not a specific indicator of a problem
Paradoxical pulse (pulsus paradoxus)	Amplitude decreases on inspiration	Chronic obstructive pulmonary disease, constrictive pericarditis, pericardial effusion
Pulsus differens	Unequal pulses between left and right extremities	Impaired circulation, usually from unilateral local obstruction
Tachycardia	Rate over 100 bpm	Fever, hyperthyroidism, anemia, shock, heart disease, anxiety, exercise
Trigeminal pulse (pulsus trigeminus)	Three beats followed by a pause	Often benign, such as after exercise; cardiomyopathy; severe ventricular hypertrophy; severe aortic stenosis; dysfunctional right ventricle
Water-hammer pulse (Corrigan pulse)	Jerky pulse with full expansion followed by sudden collapse	Aortic regurgitation

From Seidel HM et al: *Mosby's guide to physical examination*, ed 3, St Louis, 1995, Mosby.

Step	Normal/Individual Variations/Deviations
	DEVIATIONS: 140/90 mm Hg and above, coupled with evidence of end-organ damage, left ventricular hypertrophy, diabetes mellitus, smoking history, or family history of hypertension; less than 90 mm Hg systolic or 60 mm Hg diastolic; excessively wide or narrow pulse pressure; greater than 10 mm Hg difference in pressures between arms
With client standing, measure blood pressure in both arms	Drop of 10 to 15 mm Hg systolic and 5 mm Hg diastolic
	DEVIATIONS: Drop greater than 15 mm Hg systolic, 5 mm Hg diastolic, and/or symptoms of dizziness
Assess for arterial insufficiency (see Table 12-4) **Technique:** With client lying down, raise both legs about 60 degrees. Ask client to alternately flex and extend feet for about 1 minute, then sit up with legs dangling down.	Slight pallor as client moves feet; normal color returns in about 10 seconds
	Filling of veins in feet and ankles in about 15 seconds
	DEVIATIONS: Marked pallor of one or both feet; delayed color return or mottled appearance; marked dusky redness or cyanosis of dependent feet
Inspect extremities for signs of venous insufficiency (see Table 12-4): 1. Thrombosis **Technique:** With client's knee slightly flexed, acutely dorsiflex client's foot to assess calf pain response.	No pain
	DEVIATIONS: Pain (Homans' sign); redness, thickening, and tenderness along a superficial vein

Step	Normal/Individual Variations/Deviations
2. Edema **Technique:** Press index finger over bony prominence of tibia for several seconds and note depression. Measure depth of depression by grading 1^+ through 4^+ (see Fig. 12-6)	Absent, or depression refills rapidly. DEVIATIONS: Unilateral or bilateral pitting edema; skin thickening, ulceration, and pigmentation indicate deep venous obstruction or valvular incompetence
3. Varicose veins	Dilated, tortuous veins seen when legs are in dependent position; veins collapse with elevation of limbs

Continued

Table 12-4   Comparison of arterial and venous insufficiency

Arterial	Venous
Pain (claudication) comes on quickly with exercise, quickly relieved by rest; occurrence increases with intensity and duration of exercise	Pain comes on during or several hours after exercise, relieved by rest but in variable periods of time; can be constant; frequently occurs after lying flat in bed at night
Pale color when elevated, dusky red color when dependent	Skin reddish brown or cyanotic when dependent
Cool temperature	Normal temperature
Decreased or absent peripheral pulses	Normal pulse
Little or no edema	Varying degrees of edema, but usually marked from foot to calf
Thin, shiny skin with decreased hair growth; thickened nails	Hyperpigmentation; lichenification

Step	Normal/Individual Variations/Deviations
	Incompetent veins may appear as nodular bulges
	DEVIATIONS: Distended veins in anteromedial aspect of thigh and lower leg or on posterolateral aspect of calf from knee to ankle

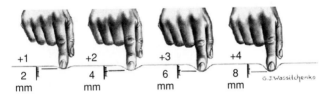

Fig. 12-6 Assessing for pitting edema.

The severity of edema may be characterized by grading 1+ through 4+. Any concomitant pitting can be mild or severe, as evidenced by the following:

1+: slight pitting, no visible distortion, disappears rapidly

2+: a somewhat deeper pit than in 1+, but again no readily detectable distortion, and it disappears in 10 to 15 seconds

3+: the pit is noticeably deep and may last more than a minute; the dependent extremity looks fuller and swollen

4+: the pit is very deep, lasts as long as 2 to 5 minutes, and the dependent extremity is grossly distorted

REMINDER: If edema is unilateral, suspect the occlusion of a major vein. If edema occurs without pitting, suspect arterial disease and occlusion. (From Seidel HM et al: *Mosby's guide to physical examination*, ed 3, 1995, Mosby.)

Step	Normal/Individual Variations/Deviations
Assess jugular venous pressure (JVP) **Technique:** Position client with head slightly elevated (30 to 45 degrees) on a pillow, sternocleido-mastoid muscle relaxed. Illuminate area with tangential light, and inspect both sides of the neck for the internal jugular vein pulsations. Be careful not to confuse the carotid artery pulsations with the venous pulsation (Table 12-5). With a centimeter ruler, measure the vertical distance between Louis's angle and the highest point of jugular vein pulsation on both sides. A straight edge of some kind intersecting the ruler at a right angle promotes accurate measurement. Record this measurement in centimeters as the JVP (Fig. 12-7).	JVP 3 cm or less DEVIATIONS: JVP over 3 cm; unilateral or bilateral distention of internal jugular veins

Continued

Table 12-5   Differentiation of the jugular and carotid pulse waves

	Jugular	Carotid
Quality and Character	Three positive waves in normal sinus rhythm	One wave
Palpate the carotid artery on one side of the neck and look at the jugular vein on other side to tell the difference	More undulating than carotid pulse	Brisker than jugular pulse
Effect of Respiration	Level of pulse wave decreased on inspiration and increased on expiration	No effect
Effect of Changing Position	More prominent when recumbent; less prominent when sitting	No effect
Venous Compression	Easily eliminates pulse wave	No effect
Apply gentle pressure over vein at base of neck above clavicle		
Abdominal Pressure	May cause some increased prominence even in healthy persons; with right-sided failure, jugular vein may be more visible	No effect
Place the palm moderately firmly over the right upper quadrant of the abdomen for half a minute		

Step	Normal/Individual Variations/Deviations
Assess hepatojugular reflux **Technique:** With client positioned as described for JVP assessment, apply moderately firm pressure using the palm of the hand for 30 to 60 seconds over the right upper quadrant of the abdomen, and note jugular vein distention.	Slight transient rise in JVP DEVIATIONS: JVP increase more than 1 cm or sustained rise in JVP

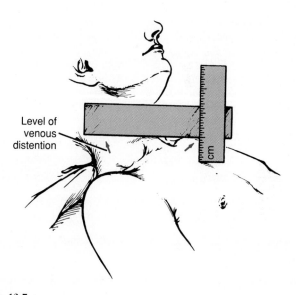

Level of venous distention

Fig. 12-7
Measure of jugular venous pressure. (From Malasanos L et al: *Health assessment,* ed 4, St Louis, 1990, Mosby.)

Continued

Step	Normal/Individual Variations/Deviations
Inspect anterior chest wall for contour, pulsations, lifts or heaves, retractions **Technique:** With tangential light illuminating client's chest, stand at client's right side and observe at eye level.	Overall symmetric contour is 2 cm or less; visible apical impulse in fifth left intercostal space at midclavicular line, with slight retraction (occurs synchronously with carotid pulse); kyphosis and scoliosis may contribute to heart displacement DEVIATIONS: Gross asymmetry; impulse located more laterally and inferiorly; rib retraction; diffuse lifting at left sternal border
Palpate precordium at apex, left sternal border, and base **Technique:** With client supine, methodically palpate all areas using the proximal halves of four fingers held together. Only lightly touch the areas, letting the movements rise to your hands. Auscultate (Fig. 12-8): Aortic valve area (second right interspace at right sternal border) Pulmonic valve area (second left interspace at left sternal border) Second pulmonic area (third left interspace at left sternal border) Tricuspid area (fourth left intercostal space at lower left sternal border) Mitral area (at apex in fifth left intercostal space at midclavicular line)	No pulsations, heaves, or thrills DEVIATIONS: Vigorous, 2 cm or more pulsation, displaced laterally and inferiorly; diffuse lifting impulse at left sternal border or fine, rushing sensation (thrill)

Step	Normal/Individual Variations/Deviations
Technique: Eliminate any room noise. With client supine, systematically listen to the five areas, first using firm pressure with the diaphragm of the stethoscope, then using light pressure with the bell of the stethoscope. Although the areas are distinctly separate, "inch" the endpiece along rather than "jumping." In each area, assess the overall rate and rhythm, the S_1, S_2, S_3, and S_4 sounds, systole, diastole, murmurs, and other sounds.	

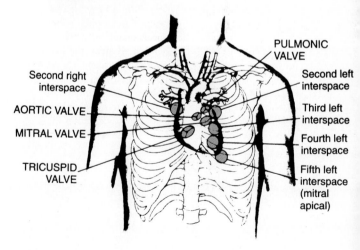

PULMONIC VALVE

Second right interspace

Second left interspace

AORTIC VALVE

Third left interspace

MITRAL VALVE

Fourth left interspace

TRICUSPID VALVE

Fifth left interspace (mitral apical)

Fig. 12-8
Areas for auscultation of the heart. (From Seidel HM et al: *Mosby's guide to physical examination,* ed 3, St Louis, 1995, Mosby.)

Continued

Step	Normal/Individual Variations/Deviations
S_1 sound	Heard at all areas but best heard at apical area; louder on the left than on the right at base; softer than S_2 on both sides of the base
	Lower in pitch than S_2 in all areas; synchronous with carotid pulse; both mitral and tricuspid components heard as one sound
	DEVIATIONS: Accentuated intensity (anemia, fever, hyperthyroidism, anxiety, mitral valve stenosis); decreased intensity (emphysema, pericardial fluid, systemic or pulmonary hypertension, fibrotic mitral valve); varying intensity (heart block, gross rhythm disruption); higher pitch with accentuated intensity
S_2 sound	Heard at all areas, but louder at the base than S_1
	Higher pitch than S_1 in all areas; shorter in duration than S_1; transient splitting at end of inspiration

Step	Normal/Individual Variations/Deviations
	DEVIATIONS: Accentuated intensity (systemic or pulmonary hypertension, mitral stenosis, congestive heart failure); decreased intensity (immobile, thickened, or calcified valves, aortic or pulmonic stenosis); wide splitting (>0.1 second on inspiration and >0.04 seconds on expiration), e.g., right bundle branch block, pulmonic stenosis, mitral regurgitation; fixed splitting (does not vary with respirations), e.g., pulmonary stenosis, right ventricular failure; paradoxical splitting (wider and more pronounced on expiration and decreased on inspiration), e.g., left bundle branch block
S_3 sound	Faint, low-pitched variable sound in early diastole, heard best at apex; may be absent
	DEVIATIONS: Accentuated intensity, particularly in left lateral position (myocardial infarction, congestive heart failure)

Continued

Step	Normal/Individual Variations/Deviations
S_4 sound	Absent DEVIATIONS: Low-pitched sound in late diastole or early systole, heard best at apex; common in the presence of hypertensive or coronary artery disease, aortic stenosis, severe anemia, or hyperthyroidism in older clients; may be indicative of myocardial ischemia
Systole	Shorter than diastole at normal heart rate DEVIATIONS: Early ejection sounds (dilated aorta, aortic valve disease, dilated pulmonary artery, pulmonary hypertension, pulmonic stenosis); clicks (mitral valve prolapse)
Diastole	Longer than systole at normal heart rate; shortens as rate increases DEVIATIONS: Pathologic S_3 or S_4
Murmurs (see Table 12-1, pp. 220-222, for summary of characteristics)	Soft, early systolic murmurs are likely "functional" and are caused by aortic lengthening, tortuosity, and sclerotic changes; diastolic murmurs are always abnormal DEVIATIONS: Loud aortic (ejection) murmurs radiating into neck may indicate obstructive aortic disease; systolic murmur at apex may indicate mitral calcification

Step	Normal/Individual Variations/Deviations
Other sounds	None **DEVIATIONS:** Pericardial friction rub: heard in all areas but loudest at apical area; occurs throughout systole and diastole, but intensity increases when client leans forward and exhales
Repeat above palpation and auscultation maneuvers with client in left lateral recumbent position and with client sitting up, leaning slightly forward	

Sample Documentation—Hypertension

Health History

Mr. B., 74, requests to have his blood pressure checked. Diagnosed with "borderline" high blood pressure 6 years ago, for which he takes HCTZ 50 mg qd. Denies weight problem, smoking; tries to follow low-salt, low-fat diet. Denies other chronic diseases; adds he has been in good health other than blood pressure problem. Denies chest pain/pressure/heaviness, SOB/DOE/PND, headache, light-headedness, edema; fatigue only when he works too long in the yard.

Physical Examination

BP 146/82 RA sitting; BP 140/80 RA standing. Apical impulse barely palpable at fifth ICS, just lateral to MCL; no lifts, heaves, or thrills palpated. S_1 and S_2 without splitting; S_1 loudest at apex, S_2 loudest as base; no S_3, S_4, or gallops. Grade II/VI holosystolic murmur heard in all areas, but best at apex. No carotid bruits. JVP wave normal, veins not distended. No edema or varicose veins BLE.

Client Teaching

Risk Factors for Cardiac Disease

1. Normal age-related changes in the heart, blood vessels, blood, and pumping ability of the heart can alter function and place the older person at risk for disease. The following risk factors for cardiac disease should be known, and, when appropriate, measures should be taken to decrease their effect.
   a. Heredity, particularly genetic predisposition for cardiovascular disease at a young age
   b. Male, black
   c. Chronic disease, especially hypertension, hyperlipidemia, and diabetes
   d. Lack of regular exercise program; sedentary life-style
   e. Diet with excessive intake of calories and fat
   f. Obesity
   g. Stress
   h. Cigarette smoking
   i. Excessive dietary intake of sodium
   j. Advanced age
2. Follow the regimen prescribed by your health care practitioner for any chronic diseases; keep follow-up appointments.
3. Develop an exercise program that you can live with. Exercise, especially walking, is very beneficial and can be readily adapted to the needs of most persons. Exercise regularly and within your level of ability. If regular exercise is coupled with dietary changes, weight reduction is possible as well.
4. Make dietary improvements; in particular, eat less saturated fats and reduce salt intake.
5. Consider enrolling in a program to stop smoking, or see your health care practitioner to discuss the use of a transdermal nicotine system.

References

Berne RM, Levy MN: *Physiology,* ed 3, St Louis, 1993, Mosby.

Malasanos L et al: *Health assessment,* ed 4, St Louis, 1990, Mosby.

National Institutes of Health: *The Fifth Report of the Joint National Committee on Detection, Evaluation, and Treatment of High Blood Pressure,* Bethesda, Md, 1993, US Department of Health and Human Services.

Seidel HM et al: *Mosby's guide to physical examination,* ed 3, St Louis, 1995, Mosby.

Thompson JM et al: *Mosby's clinical nursing,* ed 4, St Louis, 1997, Mosby.

Assessment of the Abdomen

13

The abdominal cavity contains the digestive tract and its accessory organs, as well as many vital organs of other body systems (Fig. 13-1). Symptoms relating to the gastrointestinal tract become increasingly common in older adults. Detectable, organic disease may be the cause, but sources also include nutritional intake patterns, hydration, activity, income, medications, and psychosocial problems (e.g., boredom, depression, confusion, fear, and loss). Identification of the cause of gastrointestinal symptoms requires careful assessment because both benign and serious problems frequently manifest atypically. Although age-related impairments occur in this system, the anatomic and physiologic integrity of the aging gastrointestinal tract is usually maintained.

The sequence of assessment techniques is inspection, auscultation, percussion, and palpation. Auscultation precedes percussion and palpation because manipulation of the bowel by the latter two techniques alters bowel motility and increases the incidence of sounds. Equipment needs include a stethoscope, flexible pocket ruler, and a marking pen. A strong light source, complete exposure of the abdomen from just below the breasts to the pubic area, warm hands with short fingernails, and a comfortable, relaxed client are also necessary.

For purposes of describing symptoms and examination findings, two methods of anatomic mapping are commonly used. One method divides the abdomen into four quadrants by drawing an imaginary line from the sternum to the pubis through the umbilicus, then a second horizontal line across the abdomen through the umbilicus (Fig. 13-2). The other method divides the abdomen into nine sections by drawing two imaginary vertical lines from the midclavicles to the middle of Poupart's ligament, approximating the lateral edges of the rectus abdominis muscles. At right angles

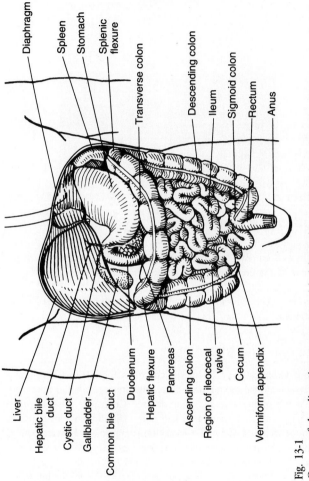

Fig. 13-1
Organs of the digestive system. (Modified from Phipps WJ et al: *Medical-surgical nursing*, ed 5, St Louis, 1995, Mosby.)

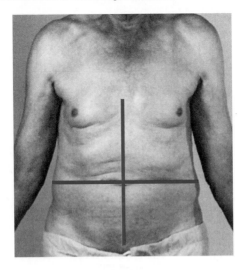

Fig. 13-2
Four quadrants of the abdomen.

to these lines, two imaginary parallel lines are drawn across the border of the costal margin and the edge of the iliac crest (Fig. 13-3). One method should be used consistently. Table 13-1 identifies the abdominal structures that correlate with the quadrants and sections.

Anatomy and Physiology

The gastrointestinal (GI) tract is approximately 30 feet long and extends from the mouth to the anus. The organs of the GI tract include the oral cavity and pharynx (see Chapter 9), esophagus, stomach, and small and large intestines. The functions of the GI tract are to ingest and digest food, absorb nutrients and water, and transport wastes for excretion. The accessory digestive organs include the liver and pancreas.

The esophagus is a collapsible muscular tube approximately 10 inches long that connects the pharynx to the stomach. Located within the mediastinum, it passes behind the trachea, through the diaphragm, and to the stomach at the cardiac orifice.

The stomach is located in the left upper quadrant immediately

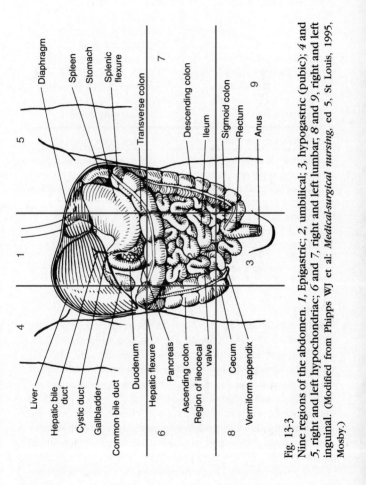

Fig. 13-3
Nine regions of the abdomen. *1*, Epigastric; *2*, umbilical; *3*, hypogastric (pubic); *4 and 5*, right and left hypochondriac; *6 and 7*, right and left lumbar; *8 and 9*, right and left inguinal. (Modified from Phipps WJ et al: *Medical-surgical nursing*, ed 5, St Louis, 1995, Mosby.)

Diaphragm
Spleen
Stomach
Splenic flexure
Transverse colon
Descending colon
Ileum
Sigmoid colon
Rectum
Anus

Liver
Hepatic bile duct
Cystic duct
Gallbladder
Common bile duct
Duodenum
Hepatic flexure
Pancreas
Ascending colon
Region of ileocecal valve
Cecum
Vermiform appendix

Table 13-1   Anatomic correlates of the four quadrants
of the abdomen

Right Upper Quadrant	Left Upper Quadrant
Liver and gallbladder	Left lobe of liver
Pylorus	Spleen
Duodenum	Stomach
Head of pancreas	Body of pancreas
Right adrenal gland	Left adrenal gland
Portion of right kidney	Portion of left kidney
Hepatic flexure of colon	Splenic flexure of colon
Portions of ascending and transverse colon	Portions of transverse and descending colon

Right Lower Quadrant	Left Lower Quadrant
Lower pole of right kidney	Lower pole of left kidney
Cecum and appendix	Sigmoid colon
Portion of ascending colon	Portion of descending colon
Bladder (if distended)	Bladder (if distended)
Ovary and salpinx	Ovary and salpinx
Uterus (if enlarged)	Uterus (if enlarged)
Right spermatic cord	Left spermatic cord
Right ureter	Left ureter

From Seidel HM et al: *Mosby's guide to physical examination,* ed 3, St Louis, 1995, Mosby.

below the diaphragm. It is a J-shaped pouch continuous with the esophagus superiorly, emptying into the duodenal portion of the small intestine inferiorly. The stomach is divided into three regions: the fundus, which is the dome-shaped portion to the left of the cardiac orifice and in direct contact with the diaphragm; the body, which is the large central portion; and the pylorus, which is the funnel-shaped terminal portion that communicates with the duodenum through the pyloric sphincter. The stomach secretes enzymes, hydrochloric acid, hormones, and mucus, which all aid digestion.

The small intestine lies between the pyloric sphincter and the ileocecal valve that opens into the large intestine, and is divided into three regions. The duodenum is a C-shaped tube about 10 inches long that receives bile secretions through the common bile duct from the liver and gallbladder and pancreatic secretions through the pancreatic duct. The jejunum is approximately 8 feet

Table 13-1   Anatomic correlates of the nine regions
of the abdomen

Right Hypochondriac	Epigastric	Left Hypochondriac
Right lobe of liver Gallbladder Portion of duodenum Hepatic flexure of colon Portion of right kidney Suprarenal gland	Pyloric end of stomach Duodenum Pancreas Portion of liver	Stomach Spleen Tail of pancreas Splenic flexure of colon Upper pole of left kidney Suprarenal gland
Right Lumbar	**Umbilical**	**Left Lumbar**
Ascending colon Lower half of right kidney Portion of duodenum and jejunum	Omentum Mesentery Lower part of duodenum Jejunum and ileum	Descending colon Lower half of left kidney Portions of jejunum and ileum
Right Inguinal	**Hypogastric (Pubic)**	**Left Inguinal**
Cecum Appendix Lower end of ileum Right ureter Right spermatic cord Right ovary	Ileum Bladder Uterus (in pregnancy)	Sigmoid colon Left ureter Left spermatic cord Left ovary

long, and it extends from the duodenum to the ileum, the 12-foot distal segment of the small intestine. The small intestine provides a large surface area for absorption of nutrients. Bile, pancreatic enzymes, and hormones aid in completing digestion.

The large intestine is structurally divided into the cecum, colon, rectum, and anal canal. The cecum is a dilated pouch that hangs inferiorly, slightly below the ileocecal valve. The appendix is a fingerlike projection attached to the cecum. The superior portion of the cecum is continuous with the colon, which consists of ascending, transverse, descending, and sigmoid portions. The ascending colon extends superiorly from the cecum along the right abdominal wall to the inferior surface of the liver. Here the colon turns sharply left at the hepatic flexure and becomes the transverse colon. Another right-angle bend called the splenic flexure is where the descending colon begins. This portion continues downward along the left abdominal wall to the pelvic region. The colon then angles medially from the rim of the pelvis to form the S-shaped sigmoid colon. The colon terminates at the rectum and anus (see Chapters 14 and 15). The primary function of the large intestine is absorption of water and the continued propulsion of its contents toward the rectum for defecation.

The liver is located in the right upper quadrant immediately beneath the diaphragm, and it extends down to the right costal margin. The liver is the largest internal organ, weighing 3.5 to 4.0 pounds, consisting of a large right lobe, a smaller left lobe, and the small quadrate and caudate lobes. These lobes are composed of lobules, the functional units of the liver. Each lobule is made up of hepatocytes surrounding a central vein. At the periphery of each lobule are branches of the portal vein, hepatic artery, and bile duct. Bile produced and secreted by the hepatocytes drains through the bile ducts into the hepatic duct, which joins the cystic duct from the gallbladder, forming the common bile duct. The liver's arterial supply is from the hepatic artery, which branches off the aorta. Foodstuffs absorbed from the stomach and intestines flow into the liver from the portal vein. Three hepatic veins from the liver drain into the inferior vena cava.

The gallbladder is a saclike organ attached to the inferior surface of the liver. This organ stores and concentrates bile, which drains to it from the liver by way of the bile ducts, hepatic duct, and cystic duct, respectively. Bile is a yellowish green fluid containing bile salts, bilirubin, and cholesterol. Bile maintains the alkaline pH of the small intestine, which permits fat absorption. The gallbladder has a storage capacity of 35 to 50 ml.

The pancreas lies retroperitoneally: the head lies in the curve of the duodenum, the body is behind the stomach, and the tail nearly touches the spleen. The pancreas has both endocrine and exocrine functions. The endocrine function is performed by the islets of Langerhans, which secrete insulin and glucagon into the blood. These hormones regulate glucose levels. Within the pancreatic lobules are the exocrine units, called acini. These cells secrete pancreatic juices that aid in the breakdown of proteins, fats, and carbohydrates.

The spleen is in the left upper quadrant, posterior and lateral to the stomach, from which it is suspended. The spleen is not a vital organ, but it does assist other organs in producing lymphocytes, filtering blood, and destroying old erythrocytes.

The two kidneys lie retroperitoneally against the back wall musculature, embedded in fat, at about the spinal cord level of T11 to L3. The right kidney is usually 1.5 to 2.0 cm lower than the left. Each kidney contains more than a million nephrons, which as the kidney's functional units are responsible for forming urine. A nephron consists of urinary tubules and associated small blood vessels. The tubular portion consists of the glomerulus, proximal convoluted tubule, loop of Henle, and distal convoluted tubule. The distal tubules of several nephrons drain into a collecting duct. The kidneys maintain the body's internal environment by excreting waste products and by regulating fluid, electrolyte, and acid-base balance via filtration, reabsorption, secretion, and excretion.

The ureters also lie retroperitoneally. Each ureter is approximately 10 inches long and begins at the pelvis of the kidney and courses inferiorly, entering the bladder at the superior lateral angle of its base. The bladder, a storage sac for urine, is located posterior to the symphysis pubis and anterior to the rectum. The urethra carries urine from the bladder to the outside of the body.

The abdominal musculature that supports and protects the abdominal cavity consists of four pairs of flat muscles: the internal oblique, external oblique, transverse abdominis, and rectus abdominis. The recti abdomini are two large muscles found on either side of the midline, extending from the anterior costal margin to the symphysis pubis. The internal and external oblique muscles and the transverse muscles form the superficial covering of the abdomen.

When the thoracic aorta penetrates the diaphragm, it becomes the abdominal aorta, which supplies blood to the abdominal organs. The main branches of the abdominal aorta are the gastric, splenic, and hepatic arteries (the celiac trunk), the superior and inferior mesenteric arteries (which supply the small intestine and colon), the renal arteries, and the common iliac arteries.

Many structural and functional changes occur in the GI tract as a consequence of aging. The motility of the esophagus, particularly in the lower third, is reduced because of the degeneration of neural cells. A condition known as achalasia results: the esophageal sphincter does not relax, and peristalsis in the esophagus is decreased or absent. The resulting dilation and delay in emptying can lead to esophageal spasm, esophagitis, and gastroesophageal reflux.

Within the stomach there is a decrease in total acid secretions, motor activity, and mucosal thickness. The decreased motor activity causes fewer hunger contractions and delayed gastric emptying. Digestive enzymes are also decreased, but enough remain available for digestion. Degeneration of gastric mucosa results in loss and degeneration of parietal cells, which in turn causes a loss of intrinsic factor necessary for vitamin B_{12} absorption. An alkaline gastric medium contributes to malabsorption of iron and thus to iron deficiency anemia.

Fewer absorbing cells, and muscular and mucosal atrophy of the small intestine, do not significantly affect structure or function. Weakened intestinal musculature and decreased peristalsis, however, do affect the large intestine. Duller nerve sensations to the lower bowel may result in a missed defecation signal, making constipation a prevalent problem. Diverticulosis, pouches on a weakened intestinal wall, is a common condition. Nausea, vomiting, flatulence, and heartburn are frequently associated symptoms.

The liver gradually decreases in size after age 50 years, which reduces its storage capacity and ability to synthesize protein. Hepatic blood flow is decreased because of a decline in cardiac output. In the absence of disease, the kidneys are able to maintain adequate fluid homeostasis despite a decline in the number of functioning nephrons. Glomerular filtration at age 90 years is about half that of a healthy 20-year-old person.

The abdomen may feel soft on palpation because of the loss of tone in the abdominal musculature; underlying organs are more easily palpated.

Assessment of the Abdomen

Equipment needed:
    Stethoscope
    Flexible pocket ruler
    Marking pen

Step	Normal/Individual Variations/Deviations
With client supine, head on small pillow, arms at sides or across chest, breasts and genitals draped, knees slightly flexed, and bladder empty, inspect:	
Skin for color, surface characteristics, scars, lesions	Color same as rest of body or slightly paler
	Smooth, soft; may have silvery white striae over lower abdomen
	Scars from surgery or trauma may be present (note location, configuration, and size on illustration of abdomen)
	(NOTE: If cause of scar was not obtained in history, inquire at this time.)
	DEVIATIONS: Jaundice, cyanosis, redness, or other discolorations; tight, shiny
	No lesions
Umbilicus for placement and contour	Centrally located
	Usually sunken but may be inverted or protrude slightly
	DEVIATIONS: Lesions, rashes; displacement upward, downward, laterally; inflammation, swelling, bulging
Contour	Flat, slightly protuberant, or scaphoid (concave)
	Increased adipose distribution overall
	DEVIATIONS: Marked distention or concavity

Continued

Step	Normal/Individual Variations/Deviations
Symmetry	Contralateral areas symmetric
	DEVIATIONS: Distention or bulges (NOTE: Mnemonic device for common causes of distention is the six Fs— fat, flatus, feces, fluids, fibroid, and fetus.)
Respiratory movement	*Male:* primarily abdominal respiratory movement
	Female: primarily costal respiratory movement
	Smooth, even movements overall
	DEVIATIONS: Respirations associated with limited or restricted movement; labored
Auscultate:	
Bowel sounds for frequency and character	Irregularly occurring clicks and gurgles at rate of 5 to 25/minute
Technique: Place warmed stethoscope on abdomen with light pressure. Use diaphragm because bowel sounds are high pitched. Develop and use a systematic route.	DEVIATIONS: Absence of sounds after 5 full minutes of listening; high-pitched tinkling; loud, gurgling borborygmi
Bruits	None
Technique: Place warm bell of stethoscope over epigastric area and all four quadrants (Fig. 13-4).	DEVIATIONS: Loud or soft, high-, medium-, or low-pitched sounds
Lower liver border (scratch test)	Sound magnified over liver
Technique: Place stethoscope over the liver while using opposite hand to lightly scratch abdominal surface with short, transverse strokes, moving toward the liver border.	

Step	Normal/Individual Variations/Deviations

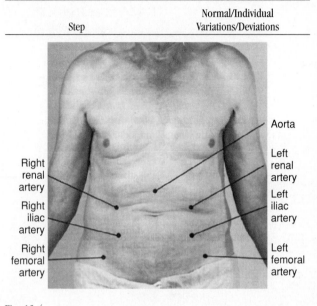

Right renal artery

Right iliac artery

Right femoral artery

Aorta

Left renal artery

Left iliac artery

Left femoral artery

Fig. 13-4
Sites to auscultate for bruits: renal arteries, iliac arteries, aorta, and femoral arteries.

Percuss:
  Four quadrants for tympany/dullness
  Technique: See Chapter 3 for review of percussion method (see Fig. 13-5 for systematic percussion route).

Predominantly tympanic over stomach and intestines
Dullness over distended bladder (suprapubic area)
DEVIATIONS: Marked dullness in any other area

Continued

Step	Normal/Individual Variations/Deviations

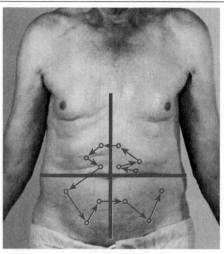

Fig. 13-5
Systematic route of abdominal percussion.

Liver span

Technique: Begin at right midclavicular line (RMCL) below umbilicus level, over area of tympany. Percuss upward along the line until dullness is heard. Mark location with pen. Now begin at RMCL over area of lung resonance. Percuss downward along the line until dullness is heard; mark that location. Measure distance between the marks to estimate span (Fig. 13-6).

Normal range is 6 to 12 cm
Lower border usually at or slightly below costal margin; upper border between fifth and seventh intercostal space (lower border may descend one or two intercostal spaces if lungs distended)

DEVIATIONS: Span greater than 12 cm or span grossly out of proportion to body size

Step	Normal/Individual Variations/Deviations

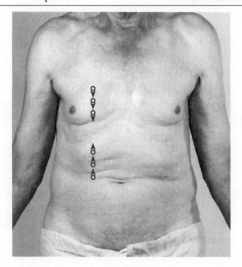

Fig. 13-6
Liver percussion route.

Spleen
Technique: Begin percussing downward just posterior to or at the left midaxillary line at the level of/or about the sixth rib to the eleventh rib (Fig. 13-7).

Small area of dullness from sixth to eleventh rib
DEVIATIONS: Dullness above sixth rib; dullness covering a large area

Stomach for gastric air bubble
Technique: Percuss in area of left lower anterior rib cage and in left epigastric region.

Lower-pitched tympany than that of the intestine
Size varies with time last meal was eaten

Continued

Step	Normal/Individual Variations/Deviations

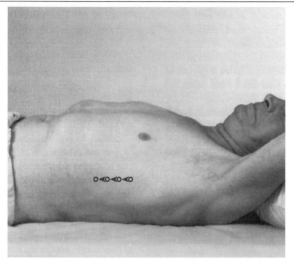

Fig. 13-7
Spleen percussion route.

Palpate:
  Four quadrants for tone, tenderness, masses
  Technique: See Chapter 3 for review of palpation method. Begin with light palpation in a systematic fashion before proceeding to deep palpation. Ask client about known areas of tenderness, and palpate those last. Mentally visualize usual placement of abdominal contents to help distinguish normal from abnormal conditions.

Lax abdominal tone; nontender during light palpation; slight discomfort over cecum, sigmoid colon, aorta, and near xiphoid
No masses; however, aorta at epigastrium and feces in ascending and descending colon may be palpable
DEVIATIONS: Involuntary resistance; guarding; localized rigidity (note location, size, shape, consistency, tenderness, pulsation, and movement with respiration if any masses palpated)

Step	Normal/Individual Variations/Deviations

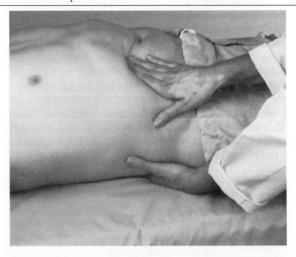

Fig. 13-8
Method for liver palpation. Fingers should be parallel to the costal margin.

Liver

Technique: Place right hand parallel to right costal margin (Fig. 13-8). Instruct client to breathe normally a few times, then take in a deep breath. At this point, gently but deeply press hand in and up. As client exhales, try to feel the liver edge as the diaphragm pushes it down to meet fingertips.

Nonpalpable, or if palpable should be firm, smooth, even, and nontender

DEVIATIONS: Enlarged, passing under hand as it extends downward

Continued

Step	Normal/Individual Variations/Deviations
Spleen	Nonpalpable, nontender
Technique: Standing at client's right side, place left hand over left costo-vertebral angle and right hand under left anterior costal margin. Palpate the spleen by pressing upward with the left hand and inward with the fingertips of the right hand as client inhales deeply (Fig 13-9).	DEVIATIONS: Palpable

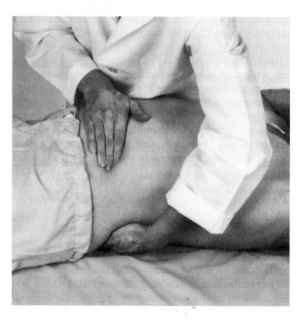

Fig. 13-9
Palpating the spleen.

Step	Normal/Individual Variations/Deviations
Kidneys **Technique:** For left kidney, stand at supine client's right side, and position left hand over client's left flank, right hand at left costal margin. Instruct client to take in a deep breath and exhale completely. As client exhales, elevate left flank with left hand, and palpate deeply with right hand (Fig. 13-10). For right kidney, place left hand under client's right flank and right hand at right costal margin. Perform same maneuvers as for the left.	Nonpalpable (lower pole of right kidney may be palpated in extremely thin client; if palpable, kidney should be smooth, firm, and nontender) DEVIATIONS: Palpable and tender

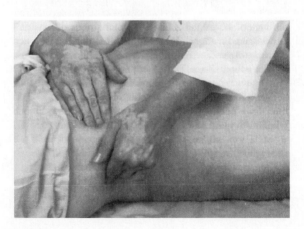

Fig. 13-10
Palpating the left kidney.

Continued

Step	Normal/Individual Variations/Deviations
Kidney tenderness **Technique:** Ask client to assume sitting position. Place palm of one hand over right costovertebral angle and strike it with ulnar surface of the fist of your other hand; repeat the maneuver over the left costovertebral angle. (NOTE: This maneuver is usually performed with posterior lung assessment for efficiency of time and client comfort.)	Nontender DEVIATIONS: Tenderness or pain
Superficial skin reflexes **Technique:** Gently stroke abdominal skin over lateral borders of rectus abdominis muscles toward the midline in each quadrant.	Brief movement of umbilicus toward side of stimulation Diminished response in obese client or in one who has sustained a good deal of abdominal stretching DEVIATIONS: Absence of reflex
Vertical and horizontal inguinal nodes for presence, contour, and consistency **Technique:** With client supine, knees slightly flexed, move fingertips of dominant hand in a gentle but probing, circular manner (see Fig. 13-11 for location).	Nonpalpable or, if palpable, small, mobile, and nontender DEVIATIONS: Enlarged, tender, fixed

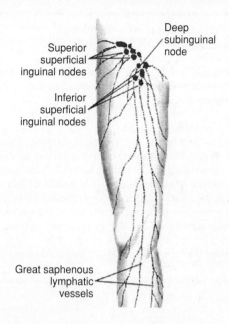

Fig. 13-11
Inguinal lymph nodes. (From Seidel HM et al: *Mosby's guide to physical examination,* ed 3, St Louis, 1995, Mosby.)

Sample Documentation—Esophageal Reflux

Health History

Miss C., 71, reports experiencing "heartburn" approximately 1 hour after most meals, but especially after her large evening meal, for about the last 2 months. Further describes it as a burning sensation between her breasts that worsens with lying down; in fact, it sometimes wakes her up at night; associated with belching and some mild regurgitation of "acidy liquid" in her mouth. Has been using 1 tsp Maalox when symptoms occur, but with little relief. Denies use of alcohol, tobacco. Drinks 4 cups coffee every morning, and 3 cola beverages daily. Denies dysphagia, abdomi-

Continued

Sample Documentation—Esophageal Reflux—cont'd

nal fullness, weight loss, diarrhea, or constipation; no bloody or tarry stools; no ho abdominal surgery. Takes no prescription drugs.

Physical Examination

Abdomen protuberant and symmetric without distention. No lesions/scars, pulsations, or visible peristalsis. Aorta in midline, pulsation barely visible; no bruit. Umbilicus centrally located, protrudes slightly. BS present all four quadrants. Renal, iliac, and femoral arteries without bruits. Tympanic percussion over epigastrium and intestines, dullness over suprapubic area. Lax abdominal tone; tenderness elicited on light and deep palpation of epigastrium. No masses. Percussed liver span 8 cm at MCL; spleen, kidneys nonpalpable. No CVA tenderness.

Client Teaching

Constipation

1. Constipation is a common condition of old age that can be managed a number of ways. It is important to remember that it can be a symptom of serious underlying disease, so if constipation does not respond to the usual self-care measures, see your health care practitioner.
2. Not everyone has a bowel movement every day, nor should this be expected. A bowel movement every 4 days or more is generally considered abnormal. If your normal bowel pattern is once every 2 to 3 days, and bowel movements are not associated with difficulty, pain, or bleeding, then you are probably not suffering from constipation.

Compiled from *Constipation,* Age Page, National Institute on Aging, Bethesda, Md, 1991, US Department of Health and Human Services, Public Health Service, National Institutes of Health.

Client Teaching—cont'd

3. The following are common, treatable causes of constipation in older persons:
   a. Inadequate fluid intake
   b. Lack of exercise or inactivity
   c. Drugs (aspirin, antihistamines, calcium channel blockers, calcium supplements, diuretics, tranquilizers, hypnotics, iron supplements, antacids with aluminum or calcium, tranquilizers, and antiparkinsonism agents)
   d. Laxative misuse or abuse
   e. Diet high in fat and refined sugar and low in fiber
   f. Neglecting to respond to the defecation urge
   g. Mental stress or depression
4. Remedies for constipation include the following:
   a. Drink at least 2 quarts of liquid/day unless contraindicated because of other health problems (heart, circulatory, or kidney problems).
   b. Participate in regular exercise; walking is a good way to keep muscles toned.
   c. Limit use of over-the-counter drugs that cause constipation, and see your health care practitioner about the possibility of changing prescribed drugs that are known to contribute to the problem.
   d. Reduce or eliminate use of laxatives, since they are habit forming and can impair the natural defecation mechanisms.
   e. Eat at least 4 servings daily of fresh fruit and vegetables, cooked or raw, and eat high-fiber foods; eat low-fat foods and reduce intake of refined sugars.
   f. Try to develop a regular elimination schedule by attempting to have a bowel movement after a meal.

References

Constipation, Age Page, National Institute on Aging, Bethesda, Md, 1991, US Department of Health and Human Services, Public Health Service, National Institutes of Health.

Phipps WJ et al: *Medical-surgical nursing,* ed 5, St Louis, 1995, Mosby.

Seidel HM et al: *Mosby's guide to physical examination,* ed 3, St Louis, 1995, Mosby.

Assessment of Male Genitalia

14

Assessment of the male genitalia includes examination of the penis; the scrotum and its contents of testicles, epididymides, and spermatic cord; the inguinal canal; the prostate gland; and the anus and rectum (Fig. 14-1). The skills of inspection and palpation are used. Gloves, lubricant, and a penlight are the only equipment needed.

Anatomy and Physiology

Penis

The penis consists of the shaft and glans penis (Figs. 14-1 and 14-2). The shaft is formed by three columns of highly vascular erectile tissue bound together by fibrous tissue: two dorsolateral columns called corpora cavernosa, and one ventromedial column called the corpus spongiosum, which contains the urethra. Erection occurs when the two corpora cavernosa and the corpus spongiosum become engorged with blood. The glans is formed by an extension of the corpus spongiosum, which surrounds the blunt ends of the corpora cavernosa. The corona is the prominence formed where the glans joins the shaft. The urethral meatus is a slitlike opening located just ventral on the tip of the glans (Figs. 14-1 and 14-2). The skin of the penis is thin, hairless, more darkly pigmented than body skin, and only loosely connected to the internal parts of the organ. Near the corona, a skinfold is formed, the prepuce or foreskin, which covers the glans. During circumcision the foreskin is removed.

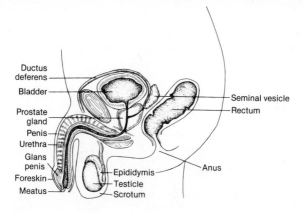

Fig. 14-1
Male sex organs. (From Potter PA: *Pocket guide to health assessment,* ed 3, St Louis, 1994, Mosby.)

Scrotum

The scrotum, also more darkly pigmented than body skin, is a loose, wrinkled pouch located at the base of the penis. The scrotum is internally divided by a septal fold of the dartos muscle into two pendulous sacs, each of which contains a testicle, epididymis, and spermatic cord (Fig. 14-3).

The ovoid-shaped testicle measures approximately 4 × 3 × 2 cm and is suspended vertically, slightly forward in the scrotum. The two primary functions of the testicles are sperm production and testosterone production.

The epididymis is a comma-shaped structure located along the posterolateral aspect and upper end of the testicle. The primary function of the epididymis is maturation, storage, and transport of sperm. The vas deferens is a duct that begins at the tail of the epididymis, ascends the spermatic cord, and passes through the inguinal canal, eventually to the side of the urinary badder. The spermatic cord comprises the vas deferens, arteries and veins, nerves, lymph vessels, and connective tissue. The inguinal canal is a 4 to 6 cm, tunnel-like opening for the spermatic cord to traverse.

The terminal portion of the vas deferens, called the ampulla, joins the ejaculatory duct. The ejaculatory duct is formed by the union of the ampulla of the vas deferens and the duct of the semi-

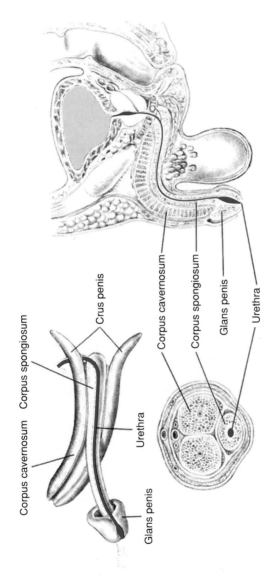

Fig. 14-2
Anatomy of the penis. (From Seidel HM et al: *Mosby's guide to physical examination*, ed 3, St Louis, 1995, Mosby.)

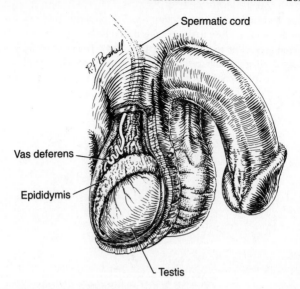

Fig. 14-3
Scrotum and scrotal contents. (From Malasanos L et al: *Health assessment,* ed 4, St Louis, 1990, Mosby.)

nal vesicle. The ejaculatory duct then pierces the prostate gland, continues through it, and empties into the urethra.

With advancing age, testosterone production declines, resulting in a slight decrease in testicular size and firmness. A gradual decrease in sperm production and in volume and viscosity of seminal fluid occurs. The scrotum becomes more pendulous because of loss of muscular tone, which may lead to trauma or excoriation of the surface.

Prostate Gland

The prostate gland is approximately 4 × 3 × 2 cm in dimension and is positioned immediately below the urinary bladder so that it surrounds the beginning of the urethra. The gland is enclosed by a fibrous capsule, and it is divided into the right and left lateral lobes and the median lobe. The median lobe enlarges with advancing age (benign prostatic hypertrophy), causing constriction of the urethra and difficulty with micturition. The posterior surface of the median lobe is close to the rectal wall and is the only portion of the gland accessible to examination (Fig. 14-4). The prostate feels enlarged, smooth, rubbery, and symmetric on palpation. The prostate secretes the enzyme acid phosphatase, which is measured clinically to assess prostate function.

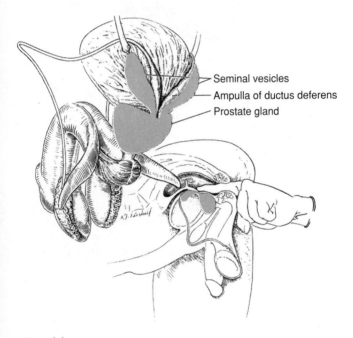

Seminal vesicles
Ampulla of ductus deferens
Prostate gland

Fig. 14-4
Prostate gland and seminal vesicles. Prostate examination. (From Barkauskas VH et al: *Health and physical assessment,* ed 2, St Louis, 1998, Mosby.)

Anus and Rectum

The anus and rectum form the terminal portion of the lower GI tract. The anal canal is a muscular sphincter 2.5 to 4.0 cm long, beginning at the anus, where the perianal skin joins the moist epithelium of the canal, and ending at the rectal ampulla, a dilation that marks the end of the large intestine. The prostate gland lies just anterior to the ampulla. The anal canal is surrounded by the internal and external sphincters, which hold it in the closed position except during elimination.

Columns of mucosal tissue, or columns of Morgagni, line the anal canal. Spaces between these columns are crypts, which exude mucus when compressed by feces. Fistulae, or fissures, may form in inflamed crypts. Crossing the columns are anastomosing veins, which form a ring known as the zona hemorrhoidalis. Dilation of these veins results in internal hemorrhoids. The lower section of the anal canal contains a venous plexus that drains downward into the inferior rectal veins. Varicosities of this plexus result in external hemorrhoids.

The rectum lies anterior to the sacrum and superior to the anus. It is approximately 12 cm long and is lined with columnar epithelium. Superiorly, the rectum is continuous with the sigmoid colon. The distal end of the rectum dilates to form the rectal ampulla, which serves as a storage place for flatus and feces. The rectal wall has three transverse folds called Houston's valves. The function of these valves is unclear, but the lowest can sometimes be palpated on examination.

Afferent neurons in the rectal wall degenerate with advancing age. Consequently, relaxation of the internal sphincter in response to fullness of the rectum is inhibited. This change is a contributing factor to constipation in old age. Rectal polyps are likely to occur in older persons and may be palpable on rectal examination, but proctoscopy is generally required and biopsy is performed to distinguish them from a malignant mass. Hemorrhoids may have developed earlier in life, or they may be a recent occurrence.

Assessment of Male Genitalia

Equipment needed:
  Gloves
  Lubricant
  Penlight

Step	Normal/Individual Variations/Deviations
With client lying or standing, inspect genital hair distribution	Thin and sparse, possible pubic alopecia Gray, straight DEVIATIONS: Patchy loss of hair
Penis	
Inspect surface characteristics	Hairless, wrinkled; dorsal vein may be evident *Circumcised:* foreskin absent; dry, smooth, pink glans without smegma DEVIATIONS: Inflammation, edema, lesions; more than slight amount of smegma
Technique: Retract or ask client to retract foreskin; it should retract easily and return to original position with ease.	*Uncircumcised:* foreskin present; moist, smooth, pink glans with slight amount of smegma DEVIATIONS: Unable to retract foreskin; painful retraction
Inspect urethral meatus	Central position at tip of glans
Technique: Compress the glans anteroposteriorly between thumb and forefinger, or ask client to compress.	Pink, glistening, without discharge DEVIATIONS: Dorsal or ventral position; redness, discharge
Palpate shaft	Soft, nontender, without nodules
Technique: Firmly compress at base of penis with thumb and forefinger, and move toward glans.	DEVIATIONS: Swelling, tenderness, localized areas of hardness

Step	Normal/Individual Variations/Deviations
Scrotum and Testes	
Inspect surface characteristics **Technique:** Ask client to hold penis out of the way.	Variations in pigmentation, but slightly darker than body skin; pendulous with fewer rugae; left side lower than right side Slight thickening (edema) resulting from general fluid retention associated with cardiac, renal, or hepatic disease DEVIATIONS: Rashes, excoriations, lesions, pitting edema
Palpate each half of scrotum simultaneously **Technique:** Gently palpate testicles, epididymis, and vas deferens between thumbs and first two fingers (note size, shape, consistency, tenderness).	*Testicles:* Slightly smaller than adult size but equal, smooth, freely movable, soft, without nodules, slightly sensitive to compression DEVIATIONS: Enlarged, grossly atrophied, nodular, fixed, tender *Epididymides:* On posterolateral surface, comma shaped, smooth, discrete, nontender DEVIATIONS: Irregular, enlarged, nodular, tender *Vas deferens:* Smooth, discrete, cordlike, nontender DEVIATIONS: Thickened, lumpy, tortuous, tender
Transilluminate each half if mass is identified or if irregularity is suspected **Technique:** Darken room, and place penlight behind scrotal contents. Transillumination casts a red glow. Serous fluid transilluminates; tissue and blood do not.	

Continued

Step	Normal/Individual Variations/Deviations
Inspect and palpate inguinal ring and canal for hernia **Technique:** With client standing and examiner sitting, or with client lying down and examiner standing at client's side, ask client to bear down as if having a bowel movement. Inspect for obvious bulging. Ask client to relax. To palpate, the index or little finger of right hand, palm side out, is used to examine a client's right side. Gently invaginate scrotal skin on right side, starting low on the scrotum. Follow spermatic cord up to inguinal ring and through canal—*do not force.* Have client cough or strain. Repeat procedure for left side.	No bulging DEVIATIONS: Bulging at area of inguinal ring or femoral area; bulging felt on fingertip, then the bulge withdraws

Anus and Perianal Area

Place client in Sims' position or with torso prone across examination table, hips flexed, feet on floor. Illuminate area with penlight.	
Inspect skin and surface characteristics	Smooth, uninterrupted skin over perianal area Coarse skin with slightly increased pigmentation of anus

Step	Normal/Individual Variations/Deviations
	DEVIATIONS: Bulges or lumps, rashes, inflammation, excoriation, pilonidal dimpling; lesions, skin tags, fissures, hemorrhoids
Palpate rectum **Technique:** Lubricate gloved index finger and press pad of finger against anal opening. As external sphincter relaxes, slip fingertip into anal canal. Ask client to strain and note external sphincter tone.	Sphincter tightens evenly around finger, no discomfort to client; very slightly lax sphincter DEVIATIONS: Grossly lax or extremely tight sphincter; tenderness, pain
Rotate finger to palpate deep external sphincter	Smooth, even pressure exerted on finger DEVIATIONS: Nodules or irregularities
Insert finger farther to palpate rectal walls	Smooth, even, uninterrupted DEVIATIONS: Nodules, masses, irregularities, polyps, tenderness
Palpate prostate, noting size, contour, consistency, and tenderness **Technique:** Rotate finger so it is in contact with anterior rectal wall to palpate posterior surface of prostate. Inform client that he may feel the urge to urinate but will not.	4 cm diameter with less than 1 cm protrusion into rectum (See box, p. 276) Median sulcus may or may not be palpable; symmetric lobes Firm, smooth consistency Nontender DEVIATIONS: Enlarged; boggy or rubbery consistency; hard and nodular; tender
Slowly withdraw finger and inspect for any fecal material, blood, or mucus; test fecal material for blood using a chemical guaiac procedure	Soft to slightly firm stool, brown DEVIATIONS: Black, tarry stool, blood or mucus, or light tan or gray stool

Sample Documentation—Benign Prostatic Hypertrophy

Health History

Mr. H., 67, reports several-month history of progressively weakening urinary stream, difficulty initiating stream, increasing frequency of urination associated with a feeling of incomplete emptying, dribbling, and nocturia four to six times/night. Denies hematuria, burning, urgency.

Physical Examination

Perianal hygiene good, without lesions, rashes, excoriation, or scars. Few small external hemorrhoidal tags. Sphincter tightens evenly; rectal walls smooth, without nodules or irregularities. Prostate: lateral lobes smooth, rubbery, and symmetric, with grade III protrusion; no nodules; sulcus not palpable. Soft brown stool, guaiac negative.

Grades of Prostatic Enlargement

Grade I	Less than 1 cm protrusion into rectal wall
Grade II	1 to 2 cm protrusion into rectal wall
Grade III	2 to 3 cm protrusion into rectal wall
Grade IV	Greater than 3 cm protrusion into rectal wall

References

Barkauskas VH et al: *Health and physical assessment,* ed 2, St. Louis, 1998, Mosby.

Malasanos L et al: *Health assessment,* ed 4, St Louis, 1990, Mosby.

Potter PA: *Pocket guide to health assessment,* ed 3, St Louis, 1994, Mosby.

Seidel HM et al: *Mosby's guide to physical examination,* ed 3, St Louis, 1995, Mosby.

Assessment of Female Genitalia

15

Assessment of the female genitalia includes examination of external genitalia, speculum and bimanual vaginal examination of internal genitalia, and rectovaginal examination. The skills of inspection and palpation are used. Equipment needs include gloves, vaginal speculum of appropriate size (Pederson is most often used with the postmenopausal client), adjustable lamp, sterile cotton-tipped applicators, spatula, glass slides, fixative, and water-soluble lubricant.

The lithotomy position required for the gynecologic examination may be difficult or uncomfortable for the older woman, depending on the degree of other body changes. For example, if the woman has cardiac or respiratory problems, elevation of the head

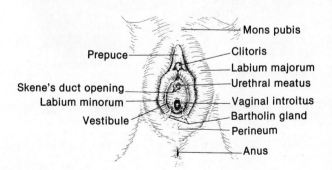

Fig. 15-1
External female genitalia. (From Bowers AC, Thompson JM: *Clinical manual of health assessment,* ed 4, St Louis, 1992, Mosby.)

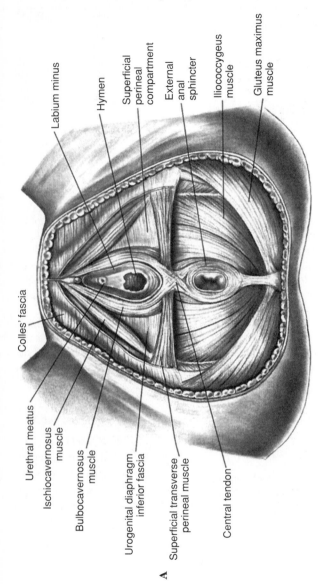

A

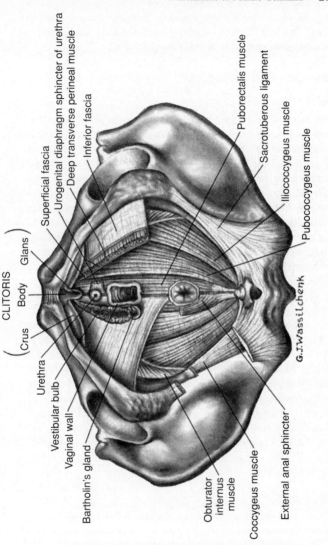

CLITORIS
Glans
Body
Crus

Superficial fascia
Urogenital diaphragm sphincter of urethra
Deep transverse perineal muscle
Inferior fascia

Puborectalis muscle
Sacrotuberous ligament
Iliococcygeus muscle
Pubococcygeus muscle

Urethra
Vestibular bulb
Vaginal wall
Bartholin's gland

Obturator internus muscle
Coccygeus muscle
External anal sphincter

G.J.Wassilchenk

B

Fig. 15-2
Musculature of the perineum. (From Thompson JM et al: *Mosby's clinical nursing*, ed 4, St Louis, 1997, Mosby.)

may facilitate breathing. Musculoskeletal changes may necessitate Sims' position. The nurse must be prepared to make adaptations as needed rather than omit the examination.

Anatomy and Physiology

External Genitalia

The external structures, collectively termed the vulva or pudendum, include the mons pubis, the labia majora and minora, the clitoris, the vestibule and its associated structures, and the perineum (Fig. 15-1). The mons pubis is a subcutaneous pad of adipose tissue covering the symphysis pubis. The labia majora are two large folds of adipose tissue lying posterior to the mons and extending to the perineum. Medial to the labia majora are two smaller skin folds, the labia minora, extending posteriorly from the clitoris to the anterior border of the perineum, forming the vaginal opening. The clitoris is an erectile structure, homologous to the penis, richly innervated with afferent endings. The clitoris is approximately 2 cm long and 0.5 cm in diameter. The vestibule is the area enclosed by the labia minora. The openings for the urethra and vagina are located here. The urethral meatus is approximately 2.5 cm behind the clitoris and immediately in front of the vaginal introitus. The vaginal opening is lubricated during sexual excitement by secretions from Bartholin's glands. Ducts from these glands open into the vestibule in the groove between the labia minora and the hymen. Multiple Skene's glands are located in the paraurethral area. Ducts draining these glands lie inside and immediately outside of the urethral meatus and may or may not be visible. The perineum is the region between the vaginal introitus and the anus. This region contains many muscles that form the pelvic floor (Fig. 15-2, *A* and *B*). Together these muscles form a sling, holding the pelvic contents in place.

Internal Genitalia

The internal organs are the vagina, the uterus, two fallopian tubes, and two ovaries (Fig. 15-3). The musculomembranous vagina is a tubelike organ about 9 cm long, passing from the cervix to the vestibule. It tilts at about a 45-degree angle, from the vaginal introitus toward the small of the back. The uterine cervix projects down into the upper end of the vagina; this creates a space around the cervix. These spaces—the anterior, posterior, and lateral fornices—have

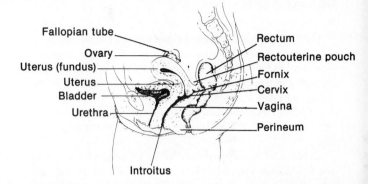

Fig. 15-3
Internal female organs. (From Bowers AC, Thompson JM: *Clinical manual of health assessment,* ed 4, St Louis, 1992, Mosby.)

thin walls through which the internal pelvic organs can be palpated.

The uterus is a hollow, thick-walled, muscular organ; it is shaped like an inverted pear; and it lies between the bladder and the rectum. It measures approximately 7 cm long, 5 cm wide, and 2.5 cm in diameter. The uppermost, dome-shaped portion, called the fundus, projects anteriorly and slightly superiorly over the bladder. The lowermost portion, the cervix, projects posteriorly and inferiorly into the vagina. The myometrium is the thick, smooth muscle layer of the uterus; the endometrium is the inner mucosal lining. The broad ligaments attach the uterus to the pelvis on both sides. The rectouterine pouch, or pouch of Douglas, is formed as the peritoneum is reflected from the uterus onto the rectum. This pouch is the lowest point in the pelvic cavity.

The fallopian tubes, or oviducts, insert in the upper portion of the uterus and run laterally toward the ovaries. Each tube is approximately 10 cm long. At the lateral end of each tube, a widened, fringed portion, the fimbria, captures the egg at ovulation.

The paired, oval-shaped ovaries are located in the upper pelvic cavity on each side of the uterus. Each ovary is about 3 cm long, 2 cm wide, and 1 cm thick. The ovaries produce eggs for release into the fallopian tubes and secrete estrogen and progesterone.

The internal genitalia are supported by the paired cardinal, uterosacral, round, and broad ligaments.

Anus and Rectum

See Chapter 14, p. 271.

The female genitalia change dramatically as a consequence of age. Because genital structures are estrogen dependent, many of these changes are associated with the cessation of ovarian estrogen production during menopause. Vulvar atrophy is caused by the resulting reduction in vascularity, elasticity, and subcutaneous fat. Consequently, it is more easily irritated. Pubic hair thins, labia majora and minora flatten and become smaller, and the introitus constricts.

Lichen sclerosus et atrophicus (LSA), a type of vulvar dystrophy, is a chronic cutaneous disease of unknown origin that may occur. Early lesions are characterized by white, flat papules with an erythematous halo and black, hard follicular plugs; in advanced cases the papules tend to coalesce into large or ivory-colored patches of thin, smooth, white, atrophic, and wrinkled skin on the vulvar area. The anogenital region is often involved as well. Mild to moderate vulvar itching and burning occur frequently.

Thinning, atrophy, and decreased vascularity of vaginal epithelium occur. The vagina shortens and narrows; becomes thin, pale, and dry; has fewer rugae; and loses elasticity and tone. Vaginal flora changes, and the environment becomes more alkaline. These alterations combine to predispose the older woman to vaginitis, dyspareunia, bleeding, cystocele, rectocele, and uterine prolapse.

Both the uterus and ovaries atrophy and may feel smaller on palpation. The cervix shrinks and appears to be thick and glistening. Loss of elasticity and tone of pelvic ligaments and connective tissue result in decreased support of pelvic contents.

Assessment of Female Genitalia

Equipment needed:
  Gloves
  Vaginal speculum
  Adjustable lamp
  Sterile, cotton-tipped applicators
  Spatula
  Glass slides
  Fixative
  Water-soluble lubricant

NOTE: Before the start of the examination:
1. Ensure that client has recently emptied bladder.
2. Have equipment within easy reach.
3. Adjust light for good visualization.
4. Warn client that you are going to touch her (with both hands gloved).

Step	Normal/Individual Variations/Deviations
External Examination	
With client in dorsolithotomy or Sims' position and examiner seated, inspect	
Hair pattern	Thin, sparse, gray, straight, but still in inverted triangular pattern
	DEVIATIONS: Patchy hair loss, absence of hair
Characteristics of mons pubis and labia majora	Flattened mons and labial folds
	Symmetric
	DEVIATIONS: Lesions, nodules, or inflammation; gross asymmetry
Inner surface of labia majora and minora (NOTE: Retract tissues gently.)	Shiny, pale, dry
	Symmetric
	DEVIATIONS: Inflammation, lesions, or nodules; gross asymmetry
Clitoris	Size variable, but usually smaller than young adult
	DEVIATIONS: Gross enlargement or atrophy; inflammation
Urethral meatus	Slitlike opening in midline, same color as surrounding tissue
	May be somewhat larger than that of young adult, and slightly more posterior, but still near or just within introitus

Continued

Step	Normal/Individual Variations/Deviations
	Ductal openings of Skene's glands and Bartholin's glands may or may not be visualized
	DEVIATIONS: Erythema, discharge, polyp
Introitus	Appearance depends on condition of hymen and parity; may be smaller than young adult or gaping if multiparous
	DEVIATIONS: Inflammation, discharge, lesions; uterine prolapse may result in bulging of mucosal tissue through opening
Perineum	Dark pink to pale pink, slightly moist to dry; evidence of scarring from lacerations or episiotomies may be visible
	DEVIATIONS: Inflammation; fistula
Palpate	
Skene's duct openings	No discharge from ducts
Technique: Separate labia majora and minora with left thumb and index finger, palm of hand resting over mons pubis. Tell client you are going to insert finger in vagina. Insert right index finger or right index and middle fingers into vagina, up to the second joint. Palm is facing upward while exerting firm, upward pressure; milk the glands in an anterior direction, moving finger(s) outward.	Nontender DEVIATIONS: Discharge; tenderness

Step	Normal/Individual Variations/Deviations
Bartholin's glands area **Technique:** Continue labial separation described above, with right index finger still in vaginal introitus. Place right thumb on lateral aspect of each side of labia minora while vaginal finger palpates the medial aspects.	Smooth, nontender, no discharge DEVIATIONS: Nodules, masses, tenderness, discharge
Perineum **Technique:** Remove left hand from mons pubis and labia. Keep right index finger in vaginal introitus. Place right thumb over perineum, and palpate the tissue between finger and thumb.	Thick and smooth in nulliparous woman, thin and rigid in multiparous woman Nontender DEVIATIONS: Lesions, growths, fistula; tenderness
Inspect for bulging and urinary incontinence **Technique:** Place right index and middle fingers in vagina and spread them laterally. Ask client to bear down.	No bulging or slight outward roll of vaginal wall Continence DEVIATIONS: Pouching of anterior wall (cystocele); pouching of posterior wall (rectocele); cervix visible at introitus or beyond (uterine prolapse); urinary incontinence (see Appendix C for discussion of incontinence)

Continued

Mechanics of the Pelvic Examination

You must make a decision about which hand to insert and hold the speculum; then you must decide which will be the intravaginal hand during the bimanual examination. Once the decision is made, maintain this routine. Often the dominant hand is more efficient with speculum insertion as well as serving as the internal hand for the bimanual assessment.

The beginning examiner should become familiar with the vaginal speculum before using it in a clinical setting. The metal speculum is very different from the disposable plastic speculum. The base of the plastic speculum widens as a portion of it moves in an adjacent groove. When the base is stabilized, it goes into place with a resounding snap that often alarms both examiner and client. The metal speculum opens and stabilizes in position with the aid of twisting lever nuts and rods. It is most helpful to "play" with these instruments in advance until you feel comfortable with them.

Step	Normal/Individual Variations/Deviations

Internal Examination (see the box on p. 286)

Insert speculum

Technique: Hold lubricated speculum with index finger over the top of the proximal end of the anterior blade, with your other fingers around the handle. Tell client that she will feel you touching her. Place pads of two fingers of opposite hand just inside introitus against posterior vaginal wall, and exert downward pressure. Obliquely (at a 45-degree downward angle), insert closed speculum over your fingers. Withdraw fingers and rotate speculum to a transverse position. Bring speculum slowly upward until cervix is viewed. Lock and stabilize speculum, open the blades, and adjust the open position of blades as needed (Fig. 15-4, *A* and *D*).

Inspect cervix for color, position, size, discharge, and surface characteristics

Pale pink color, evenly distributed; midline position; projecting 1 to 3 cm into vaginal vault; smaller than the 2 to 3 cm size of younger adult

Minimal discharge; if present, should be odorless, clear to white, and thin

Continued

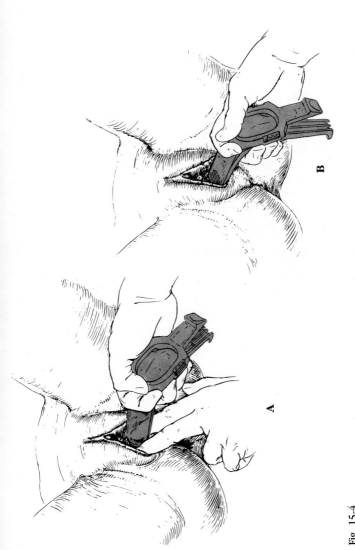

Fig. 15-4
Procedure for vaginal examination. **A,** Opening of the introitus. **B,** Oblique insertion of the speculum.

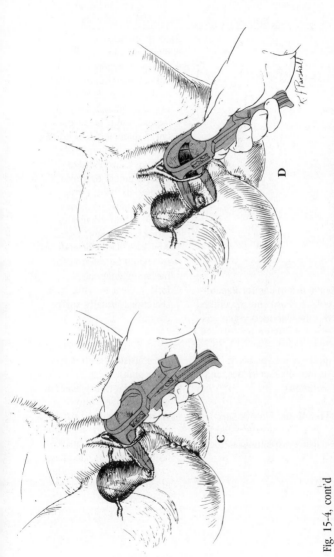

Fig. 15-4, cont'd

C, Final insertion of the speculum. **D,** Opening of the speculum blades. (From Malasanos L et al: *Health assessment,* ed 4, St Louis, 1990, Mosby.)

Step	Normal/Individual Variations/Deviations
	Smooth surface Nabothian cysts DEVIATIONS: Hyperemic, gross pallor, cyanotic; deviation to the right or left; projecting more than 3 cm into vaginal vault; larger than 4 cm in diameter; foul odor of discharge, with color varying from white to yellow, green, or gray; bloody discharge; irregular, rough, friable erosions; punctile hemorrhages or "strawberry spots" (NOTE: Any irregularity or nodularity should be referred for further evaluation.)
Obtain specimens for Papanicolaou (Pap) smear, culture, or other laboratory analysis (see the box on pp. 291-293)	Odorless, clear to white, thin secretions; usually sparse overall
Inspect vagina for color, surface characteristics, and secretions	Color consistent with cervix (pale pink) Slightly moist to dry, smooth with no rugae, shiny
Technique: Unlock speculum and slowly withdraw using a rotating motion.	DEVIATIONS: Reddened patches, lesions, or pallor; leukoplakia; markedly dry, cracked; lesions, bleeding, nodules, swelling; foul odor; yellow, green, gray, or excessive secretions

Procedures for Obtaining Vaginal Smears and Cultures

Very often during the speculum examination, you will be obtaining vaginal specimens for smears and cultures. Vaginal specimens are obtained while the speculum is in place in the vagina, but after the cervix and its surrounding tissue have been inspected. Collect the Pap smear first, followed by gonococcal and other smears as indicated. Label the specimen with the client's name and a description of the specimen (e.g., cervical smear, vaginal smear, and culture). Be sure to follow Centers for Disease Control (CDC) guidelines for the safe collection of human secretions.

Pap Smear

Brushes are now being used in conjunction with or instead of the conventional spatula to improve the quality of cells obtained. The cylindric-type brush (for example, a Cytobrush) collects endocervical cells only. First, collect a sample from the ectocervix with a spatula (see figure below). Insert the longer projection of the spatula into the cervical os. Rotate it 360 degrees, keeping it flush against the cervical tissue. Withdraw the spatula, and spread the speci-

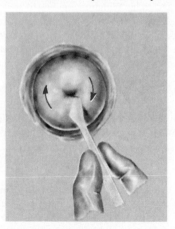

From Seidel HM et al: *Mosby's guide to physical examination,* ed 3, St Louis, 1995, Mosby.   *Continued*

Procedures for Obtaining Vaginal Smears and Cultures—cont'd

men on a glass slide. A single light stroke with each side of the spatula is sufficient to thin the specimen out over the slide. Immediately spray with cytologic fixative and label the slide as the ectocervical specimen. Then introduce the brush device into the vagina and insert it into the cervical os until only the bristles closest to the handle are exposed. Slowly rotate one-half to one full turn. Remove and prepare the endocervical smear by rolling and twisting the brush with moderate pressure across a glass slide. Fix the specimen with spray and label as the endocervical specimen. Warn the client that she may have blood spotting after this procedure. The paintbrush-type brush (for example, Cervexbrush) is used for collecting both ectocervical and endocervical cells at the same time. This brush utilizes flexible plastic bristles, which are reported to cause less blood spotting after the examination. Introduce the brush into the vagina, and insert the central long bristles into the cervical os until the lateral bristles bend fully against the ectocervix. Maintain gentle pressure and rotate the brush by rolling the handle between the thumb and forefinger three to five times to the left and right. Withdraw the brush, and transfer the sample to a glass slide with two single paint strokes: apply first one side of the bristle, turn the brush over, and paint the slide again in exactly the same area. Apply fixative and label as the ectocervical and endocervical specimen.

Gonococcal Culture Specimen

Immediately after the Pap smear is obtained, introduce a sterile cotton swab into the vagina and insert it into the cervical os. Hold it in place for 10 to 30 seconds. Withdraw the swab, and spread the specimen in a large Z pattern over the culture medium, rotating the swab at the same time. Label the tube or plate, and follow agency routine for transporting and warming the specimen. If indicated, anal culture can be obtained after the vaginal speculum has been removed. Insert a fresh, sterile cotton swab about 2.5 cm into the rectum and rotate it full circle. Hold it in place for 10 to 30 seconds.

From Seidel HM et al: *Mosby's guide to physical examination,* ed 3, St Louis, 1995, Mosby.

Procedures for Obtaining Vaginal Smears and Cultures—cont'd

Withdraw the swab, and prepare the specimen as described for the vaginal culture.

Chlamydial Enzyme Immunoassay Specimen

Collect this specimen after the gonococcal specimen if both are indicated. Remove excess mucus from the ectocervix with a separate swab and discard. Introduce the appropriate swab (provided with or specified by the kit) into the vagina. Insert into the cervical os and rotate for 15 to 30 seconds to ensure adequate sampling and absorption by the swab. Avoid touching the vaginal walls with the swab. Remove the swab and immediately place it in the transport tube containing the specimen reagent. The swab must contact the solution. Label appropriately, and follow agency procedure for testing, storage, and, if necessary, shipping. In-office test kits are now available. Conjunctival and nasopharyngeal samples can also be obtained using separate swabs. In males, a urogenital sample can be obtained. Follow procedures outlined in the kit instructions.

Dry Smear, Wet Prep, and Potassium Hydroxide Procedures

Prepare the appropriate glass slides before you obtain the specimens for these tests. For *Gardnerella (Haemophilus) vaginalis* use a dry glass slide; for *Trichomonas vaginalis,* mix the secretions with a drop of saline solution on a glass slide; and for *Candida albicans,* mix the secretions with a drop of potassium hydroxide (KOH) on a glass slide. Introduce the plain wooden end of a sterile cotton swab into the vagina, and roll it in the vaginal discharge. Withdraw the swab, and smear the secretions on the dry slide or mix the sample in 2 drops of solution using a stirring, rolling motion. Cover the glass slides with coverslips, and label the specimens. The slide is immediately examined under the microscope for characteristic clue cells of *H. vaginalis,* for trichomonads of *T. vaginalis,* or for mycelia and spores of *C. albicans.*

Step	Normal/Individual Variations/Deviations
Bimanual Examination (see Fig. 15-5)	
Technique: Move to standing position. Remove glove from one hand and lubricate index finger, or index and middle fingers, of gloved examining hand. Introduce finger(s) into vagina, in a posterior direction with palmar surface upward; thumb is abducted, third and fourth fingers are flexed into the palm and remain outside vagina.	
Palpate (as you enter)	
Vaginal wall	Smooth, homogeneous
	Nontender
	DEVIATIONS: Nodules, masses; tender
Cervix for size, shape, consistency, position, mobility, and patency of os	Smaller than young adult size of 2.5 to 4.0 cm
	Smooth and firm
Technique: Locate cervix with fat pads of fingers, and run fingers around it. Then gently palpate between your fingers and move it from side to side. Gently insert tip of one finger into os.	Midline position, pointing downward or upward
	Freely movable without discomfort
	May or may not be able to insert fingertip 0.5 cm, but os should be palpable
	DEVIATIONS: Enlarged; nodular, hard, rough; laterally displaced; fixed position, tenderness associated with movement; severe stenosis
Uterus for position, size, shape, consistency, mobility, and surface characteristics	Smaller than that of younger woman; frequently nonpalpable
	Freely movable

Continued

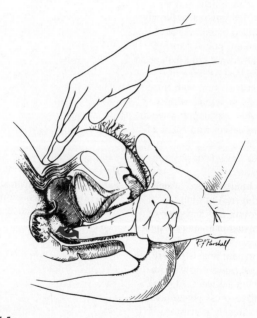

Fig. 15-5
Bimanual palpation of the uterus. (From Malasanos L et al: *Health assessment*, ed 4, St Louis, 1990, Mosby.)

Step	Normal/Individual Variations/Deviations
Technique: Place "vaginal" finger(s) in the anterior fornix. Place fingertips of other hand on abdominal midline, halfway between the umbilicus and the symphysis pubis. Slowly slide abdominal hand toward pubis, pressing downward with flattened fingers. At same time, push upward with fingertips of vaginal hand while pushing downward on cervix with backs of fingers. See Fig. 15-6, *A, C, E, G, I* for position.	DEVIATIONS: Markedly enlarged; fixed position, nodular, hard, irregular, or tender
Ovaries	Rarely palpable
	Fallopian tubes nonpalpable
Technique: Place "vaginal" finger(s) in right lateral fornix and fingertips of abdominal hand on right lower quadrant. Press vaginal fingers inward and upward toward abdominal hand. At same time, press inward and obliquely downward toward symphysis pubis with flattened fingers of abdominal hand. Palpate tissues between the two hands. Repeat maneuver on other side.	DEVIATIONS: Masses, nodules, or tenderness in adnexal area

Text continued on p. 302

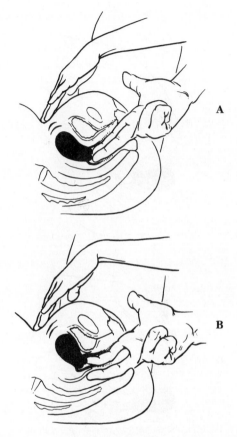

Fig. 15-6
Findings in bimanual vaginal and rectovaginal examination.
A and **B:** Anteverted uterus. **A,** Bimanual technique. Position of cervix: anterior vaginal wall. Uterine body and fundus palpable by one hand on the abdomen and the fingers of the other hand in the vagina. Anterior and posterior portion of uterus: palpable as the uterus is rotated even more anteriorly. **B,** Rectovaginal position. Cervix is palpable through the rectovaginal septum. Uterine body and fundus not palpable by fingers in the rectum. (Modified from Malasanos L et al: *Health assessment,* ed 4, St Louis, 1990, Mosby.)   *Continued*

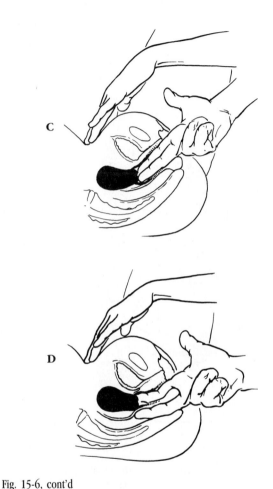

Fig. 15-6, cont'd
C and **D:** Midposition uterus. **C,** Bimanual technique. Position of cervix is at the apex of the vagina. Uterine body and fundus may not be palpable. Anterior and posterior portions of uterus may not be palpable. **D,** Rectovaginal position. Posterior portion of cervix is felt through the rectovaginal septum. Uterine body and fundus may not be palpable. (Modified from Malasanos L et al: *Health assessment,* ed 4, St Louis, 1990, Mosby.)

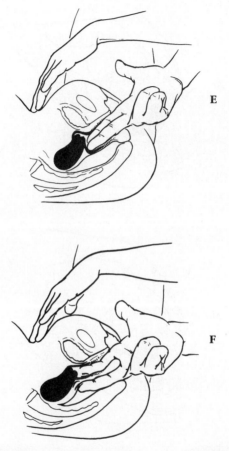

Fig. 15-6, cont'd

E and **F:** Retroverted uterus. **E,** Bimanual technique. Position of cervix: Posterior vaginal wall. Uterine body and fundus are not palpable. Posterior portion of uterus may be palpable by fingers in posterior fornix. **F,** Rectovaginal position. Cervix may not be palpable by fingers in the rectum. Uterine body is easily palpable by fingers in the rectum; fundus may not be palpable.   *Continued*

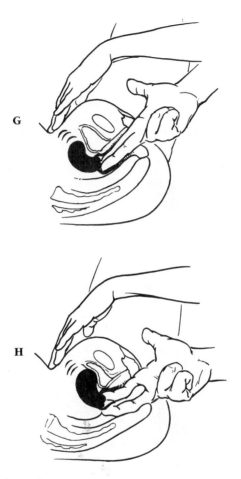

Fig. 15-6, cont'd
G and **H:** Anteflexed uterus. **G,** Bimanual technique. Position of cervix: Anterior vaginal wall or apex. Uterine body and fundus are easily palpable; angulation of the isthmus may be felt in the anterior fornix. Anterior and posterior portions of uterus are easily palpable. **H,** Rectovaginal position. Cervix palpable through the rectovaginal septum. Uterine body and fundus are not palpable by fingers in the rectum. (Modified from Malasanos L et al: *Health assessment,* ed 4, St Louis, 1990, Mosby.)

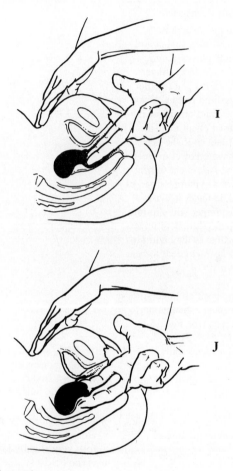

Fig. 15-6, cont'd
I and **J:** Retroflexed uterus. **I,** Bimanual technique. Position of cervix: Anterior or posterior vaginal wall or apex. Uterine body and fundus are not palpable. Anterior and posterior portions of uterus are not palpable. **J,** Rectovaginal position. Cervix is palpable through the rectovaginal septum. Angulation is palpable; uterine body and fundus are easily palpable.

Step	Normal/Individual Variations/Deviations
Rectovaginal Examination	
Technique: Withdraw fingers from vagina and change gloves. Lubricate and insert index finger into vagina and middle finger into rectum. Place other hand on abdomen. Instruct client that she will feel as if she needs to have a bowel movement. Ask client to bear down as you press pad of middle finger against anus; finger will slip into rectum. Slide both fingers in as far as they will go, and instruct client to bear down.	
Palpate	
Uterine position to confirm bimanual examination findings (see Fig. 15-6, *B, D, F, H, J*)	
Anterior rectal wall	Firm, thick, smooth, and pliable; nontender DEVIATIONS: Nodules, masses, thickening, bulging; tenderness
Anal sphincter tone (while withdrawing finger)	Sphincter tightens evenly around finger, no discomfort; very slightly lax tone DEVIATIONS: Grossly lax, or extremely tight sphincter; tenderness, pain
Test feces using a chemical guaiac procedure	
Wipe excess lubricant from vulva and anus, and assist client to sitting position	

Sample Documentation—Atrophic Vaginitis

Health History

Mrs. F., 72, reports about a 3-month duration of vulvar and vaginal burning and soreness, with occasional itching, and dyspareunia. Occasionally notes burning on urination. Denies discharge; has noticed a few episodes of light bleeding, after intercourse. Does not use bubble baths or genital deodorants. Has done nothing for relief: "I just don't know what to do, and I'm so miserable with this." Total hysterectomy at age 57 years. No history of ERT; currently taking no medications.

Physical Examination

Female hair distribution; gray and thinning. No masses, lesions, or swelling of vulva. Labia shiny, pale pink, dry. No redness, swelling, or discharge from urethral orifice or ducts/glands. Vaginal mucosa pale and shiny overall, but with a few scattered petechiae noted and an approximate 0.5 cm erosion on the posterior surface, just inside vaginal introitus; thin, sparse, watery discharge without odor. Rectovaginal septum intact without lesions. Perianal hygiene good, without lesions, rashes, or excoriations. Sphincter tightens evenly, but with slightly lax sphincter tone. Rectal walls smooth and even, without nodules/masses. Soft, dark brown stool guaiac negative.

References

Bowers AC, Thompson JM: *Clinical manual of health assessment,* ed 4, St Louis, 1992, Mosby.

Malasanos L et al: *Health assessment,* ed 4, St Louis, 1990, Mosby.

Seidel HM et al: *Mosby's guide to physical examination,* ed 3, St Louis, 1995, Mosby.

Thompson JM et al: *Mosby's clinical nursing,* ed 4, St Louis, 1997, Mosby.

Assessment of the Musculoskeletal System

16

Musculoskeletal assessment includes examination of bones, joints, and muscles. Assessment of these systems is complex because (1) they are responsible for body movement, support, and stability, and (2) their function is highly integrated with skin and neurologic systems. Data collection is further complicated because when a regional approach is used, this assessment is usually integrated with other parts of the total examination. Consequently, the nurse should have a sound knowledge of skeletal system anatomy, including joint anatomy and range of motion norms, and names and functions of major muscle groups.

Bones and their articulations, as well as muscles, undergo age-related changes that affect physical appearance and physiologic function. Coupled with multiple and varied physical, psychosocial, and environmental factors that affect mobility, assessment of the older adult is a challenging process. The nurse's skill, experience, and knowledge of gerontologic principles determine the accuracy and completeness of the assessment.

Inspection and palpation are the major techniques used as the client assumes a variety of positions. Equipment needs include a tape measure and goniometer. If possible, conduct musculoskeletal system assessment in the client's usual environment and when the client is not stressed or fatigued. Consideration must also be given to other health problems that may affect assessment, such as respiratory system disease, depression, or a long-standing poor nutritional intake. Periodic rest periods during assessment may be necessary. The extensiveness of the examination depends on the client's general condition and symptoms.

Anatomy and Physiology

The bones of the skeletal system perform the functions of support, protection, body movement, hematopoiesis, and mineral storage (Fig. 16-1). Skeletal muscle tissue attaches to the skeleton and is responsible for voluntary body movement (Fig. 16-2, *A* and *B*). Joints are classified structurally and functionally (Table 16-1). Structural classification is based on the material binding the bones together and whether or not a joint cavity is present. Functional classification is based on the amount of movement allowed at the joint. As the articulation between adjacent bones, joints hold bones together and allow movement. Joint movements are described in Table 16-2.

Osteoporosis is a progressive loss of total bone mass that occurs with aging. Some of the possible causes of this loss include physical inactivity, hormonal changes, chronic corticosteroid use, thyroid supplements, and actual bone resorption. The effect of bone loss is weaker bones: vertebrae are softer and may become compressed, and long shaft bones are less resistant to bending and thus more prone to fracture. The most common fracture sites are hip, vertebrae, and wrist. Accompanying the bone loss from the inside (endosteum) surface is an actual bone gain on the outside (periosteum) surface. Consequently, spurs and ridges form, making some bony prominences more prominent.

Skeletal muscle fibers degenerate. Fibrosis occurs as collagen replaces muscle, interfering with the attainment of oxygen and nutrient supplies. Muscle mass, tone, and strength all decrease: the more prominent muscles of the extremities become thin and flabby, and the hands grow thin and bony. Muscle rigidity increases, particularly in the extremities and neck, which diminishes ease of movement and range of motion. Shrinkage and sclerosis of tendons and muscles result in an overall delayed response during testing of deep tendon reflexes.

Calcification of the articular cartilage, coupled with noninflammatory deterioration of the weight-bearing joints, may occur. Synovial fluid thickens, and hyaline cartilage degenerates. These changes can affect range of motion, overall ease of movement, and

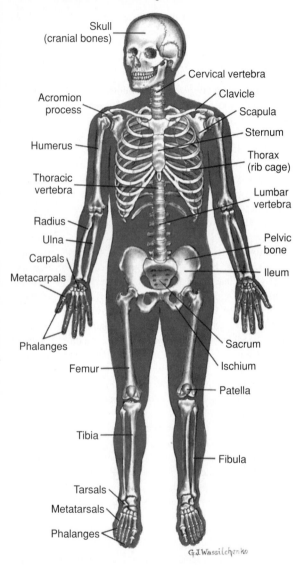

Fig. 16-1
Bones that make up the axial and appendicular skeletons.
(From Thompson JM et al: *Mosby's clinical nursing,* ed 3, St Louis, 1993, Mosby.)

Table 16-1 Classification of joints

Type of Joint	Example	Description
Synarthrosis		No movement is permitted
Suture	Cranial sutures	United by thin layer of fibrous tissue
Synchondrosis	Joint between the epiphysis and diaphysis of long bones	A temporary joint in which the cartilage is replaced by bone later in life
Amphiarthrosis		Slightly movable joint
Symphysis	Pubic symphysis	Bones are connected by a fibrocartilage disk
Syndesmosis	Radius-ulna articulation	Bones are connected by ligaments
Diarthrosis (synovial)		Freely movable; enclosed by joint capsule, lined with synovial membrane
Ball and socket	Hip	Widest range of motion, movement in all planes
Hinge	Elbow	Motion limited to flexion and extension in a single plane
Pivot	Atlantoaxis	Motion limited to rotation
Condyloid	Wrist between radius and carpals	Motion in two planes at right angles to each other, but no radial rotation
Saddle	Thumb at carpal-metacarpal joint	Motion in two planes at right angles to each other, but no axial rotation
Gliding	Intervertebral	Motion limited to gliding

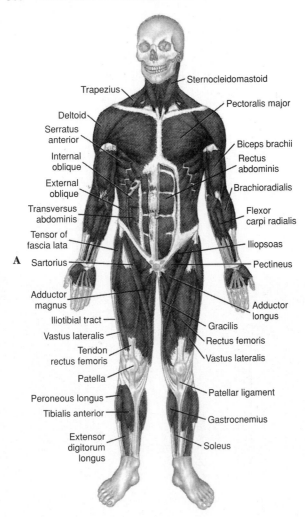

Fig. 16-2
Muscles of the body. **A,** Anterior view. (From Thompson JM et al: *Mosby's clinical nursing,* ed 4, St Louis, 1997, Mosby.)

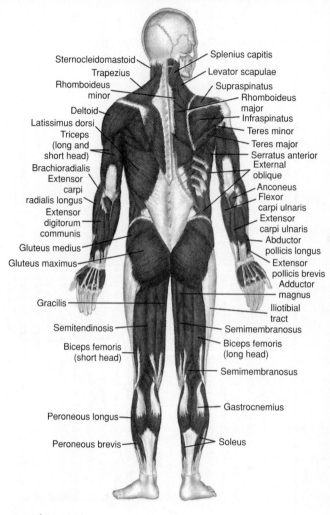

Fig. 16-2, cont'd
B, Posterior view. (From Thompson JM et al: *Mosby's clinical nursing,* ed 4, St Louis, 1997, Mosby.)

Table 16-2   Joint movement

Movement	Description
Flexion	Bending movement that decreases the joint angle on an anterior-posterior plane. EXAMPLES: Bending of elbow, knee, head.
Extension	Straightening movement (opposite of flexion) that increases the joint angle. EXAMPLES: Straightening of elbow or knee from flexion position.
Abduction	Movement of a body part away from the main axis of the body, from the midsagittal plane, or in a lateral direction.
	EXAMPLES: Moving arm upward and away from body or spreading fingers apart.
Adduction	Movement of a body part toward the main axis of the body (opposite of abduction). EXAMPLE: In the anatomic position, arms and legs are adducted toward the midplane of the body.
Rotation	Movement of a bone around its own axis. Internal rotation is turning a body part inward toward the main axis of the body; external rotation is turning the part away from the main axis. EXAMPLE: Turning head from side to side in a "no" motion.
Circumduction	Circular, conelike movement of a body segment. The distal part of the extremity actually performs the movement while the proximal attachment forms the pivot. EXAMPLE: Possible at shoulders, wrist, trunk, hip, and ankle joints.
Inversion	Movement of the sole of the foot inward, or medially.
Eversion	Movement of the sole of the foot outward, or laterally.
Pronation	Rotational movement of the forearm in which the palm of the hand is turned posteriorly.
Supination	Rotational movement of the forearm, in which the palm of the hand is turned anteriorly.

gait. Ankylosis of the ligaments and joints contributes to the picture of generalized flexion.

Foot Assessment

Although not considered to be a distinct component of traditional assessment, the feet of the older adult should be thoroughly assessed. The condition of the feet can greatly influence one's physical, psychosocial, and functional well-being, yet little attention is generally given to assessing the feet of older adults. Years of use/misuse, wear and tear, trauma, neglect, visual and/or mobility impairments, and systemic disease conditions can all lead to a variety of foot problems, including various lesions, gait difficulties, pain, and increased risk for falls. Problems identified on assessment can provide valuable clues to the older adult's well-being and functional ability.

The assessment of the feet includes inquiry about symptoms and self-care practices as well as basic inspection and palpation (see the box on pp. 311-312). The specific problems of corns, calluses, bunions, hammertoes, fissures, and nail disorders may require podiatric referral. The nurse has an important role in educating older adults about all aspects of footcare, as well as selection of proper footwear (see the box on p. 313).

Essentials of Foot Assessment

Inquire About:

Chronic diseases: diabetes mellitus, gout, osteoarthritis, rheumatoid arthritis, peripheral vascular disease, pernicious anemia, and ulcers

Conditions such as foot drop, eversion or inversion deformity, and amputations

Usual foot care practices and impairments affecting same, use of podiatrist

Activity limitations related to condition of feet

Use of mobility aids

Use and type of footwear

Use of garters or other circular constricting items

Smoking history

Fall history

Continued

Essentials of Foot Assessment—cont'd

Observe:

Mobility
Gait
Footwear
Overall hygiene

Inspect for:

Color of skin and nails
Hair growth
Edema
Pressure areas
Varicosities
Hydration
Skin lesions
Corns, calluses, bunions, hammertoes, overlapping digits, and fissures
Condition of nails, including presence of fungal nail infections
Evidence of use of home remedies

Palpate for:

Temperature
Moisture
Pulses
Capillary refill

Test for:

Sensory response to temperature, light touch, pin prick, vibration, and position

Foot Care Guidelines for Older Adults

Inspect feet daily for redness, breaks in skin, blisters. If unable to do, have someone else do it for you.

Wash with warm, not hot water, and use mild soap; test temperature of water with hand or elbow.

Blot dry only, and dry carefully between toes.

Apply emollient lotion to skin that is thoroughly dry, but not between toes.

Use a pumice stone, a little each day, on corns and calluses after washing feet.

Soak brittle nails before trimming for 15 to 20 minutes in warm, not hot water.

Trim toenails straight across and even with the tips of toes; never cut the corners.

Avoid use of razors or over-the-counter preparations for corns and calluses.

Obtain the services of a podiatrist for nails that are extremely thick, or for corns and calluses that are resistant to treatment with a pumice stone.

Wear clean socks or stockings every day; wear cotton socks when possible.

Avoid use of garters, trousers socks or knee-high stockings with tight elastic bands, or knotted stockings.

Check inside of shoes visually and with fingers for roughened areas and foreign bodies before putting on feet.

Never walk barefoot; wear slippers when getting up at night.

Avoid extremes of temperature, especially heating pads and hot water bottles.

Do not smoke.

Notify health care professional immediately of any injuries or lesions.

Purchase new shoes at the end of the day, when feet may be swollen; break in gradually; look for shoes with the following characteristics:

Wider toe box, a little longer

Snug-fitting heel

Flexible sole that grips slippery surfaces

Comfortable arch support

Cushioning devices inside for comfort and shock absorption

Assessment of the Musculoskeletal System

Equipment needed:
   Tape measure
   Goniometer

NOTE: Client should be sufficiently exposed to conduct careful and complete observations; however, give consideration to overall warmth, modesty, and comfort.

Step	Normal/Individual Variations/Deviations
At the start of the assessment, inspect	
Overall body symmetry, alignment of extremities, any gross deformities, and posture	Symmetry of body parts; slight asymmetries may be of no pathologic significance
	Extremities aligned, with contour, symmetry, and angles bilaterally equal; extremities appear long because trunk size has diminished
	Overall appearance is one of general flexion: head and neck thrust forward; dorsal kyphosis; flexion at elbows, wrists, hips, and knees; wide-based stance
	DEVIATIONS: Gross asymmetry or deformities; varus deformity (bowlegs), valgus deformity (knock-knees); lordosis, scoliosis
Muscles for gross hypertrophy or atrophy	Wasting may be found near mobility-restricted joints; guttering in the intercarpal grooves; overall limb appearance is oval, with flattened sides in the anterior and posterior position when limb is in horizontal position; asymmetry of 1 cm or less

Step	Normal/Individual Variations/Deviations
	DEVIATIONS: Gross hypertrophy or atrophy
Palpate bones, joints, and muscles for swelling, tenderness, localized temperature changes, and crepitation	Absent to slight swelling and/or tenderness, depending on history
	Temperature generally equal throughout
	No crepitation
	DEVIATIONS: Gross prominences, swelling, or tenderness (NOTE: If swelling is fluctuant, it is due to fluid; if firm, it is caused by thickening or enlargement); hot or cold in comparison to rest of body; crepitation with movement; fasciculations
Assess muscle strength	See Table 16-3 for muscle strength grading scale; muscle strength greater in dominant arm or leg
NOTE: Evaluation of strength of muscle groups from head to toe is incorporated with assessment of range of motion. Techniques for muscle strength screening tests are as follows:	DEVIATIONS: Grade 3 or less indicates disability that may impair functional ability
Technique (ocular musculature): Attempt to open client's eyelids as client keeps lids tightly closed.	
Technique (facial musculature): Place fingers on client's cheek and assess pressure against cheek bulge created as client blows out cheeks.	
Technique (neck musculature): Place hand on client's upper jaw as client turns head laterally against resistance.	

Continued

Table 16-3 Scale for grading muscle strength

Functional Level	Lovett Scale	Grade	Percentage of Normal
No evidence of contractility	Zero	0	0
Evidence of slight contractility	Trace	1	10
Complete range of motion with gravity eliminated	Poor	2	25
Complete range of motion with gravity	Fair	3	50
Complete range of motion against gravity with some resistance	Good	4	75
Complete range of motion against gravity with full resistance	Normal	5	100

From Malasanos L et al: *Health assessment,* ed 4, St Louis, 1990, Mosby.

Step	Normal/Individual Variations/Deviations
Technique (shoulder musculature): Place hand over client's shoulder at about midclavicular line as client raises shoulders against resistance.	
Technique (deltoid musculature): Place hands over client's deltoid muscles with client's arms abducted to 90 degrees; have client hold position against resistance.	
Technique (biceps): Place pressure on client's fully extended forearm as client tries to flex arm.	
Technique (triceps): Place pressure on client's flexed forearm as client tries to extend arm.	

Step	Normal/Individual Variations/Deviations
Technique (wrist and finger musculature): Place hand over palm of client's fully extended hand as client tries to flex wrist against resistance.	
Technique (hip musculature, supine): Place hand over client's slightly raised and extended leg as client tries to hold it up against resistance.	
Technique (quadriceps, sitting): Place hand over client's stiffly extended leg and attempt to flex it.	
Technique (hamstring, sitting): Place hands behind client's tightly flexed lower extremity and attempt to extend it.	
Technique (ankle and foot musculature): Place hand on dorsal surface of client's neutrally positioned foot as client attempts to bend foot up against resistance.	
Assess range of motion for joints listed in Table 16-4, using these principles: 1. Symmetry is the key. 2. Develop and use a consistent approach. 3. Consider the effect of findings on the client's functional ability. 4. Observe facial expression for indication of pain or discomfort.	Refer to Table 16-4 DEVIATIONS: Range of motion significantly below normal and affecting functional ability.

Continued

Table 16-4   Range of motion assessment

Joint	Motion and Client Instructions	Measurement*
Temporomandibular	Open and close mouth.	3 to 6 cm between teeth
	Move jaw from side to side.	1 to 2 cm mandibular movement in each direction
Cervical spine	Move jaw forward, then backward.	Expect both movements
	Flexion: Bend head forward, and touch chin to chest.	45°
	Extension: Bend head backward with chin toward ceiling.	55°
	Lateral bending: Bend head to each side, and touch ear to shoulder.	40° to right and left
	Rotation: Turn head, and touch chin to shoulder.	70° right to left
Lumbar spine	*Flexion:* Bend forward at the waist.	75° to 90°
	Extension: Bend backward at the waist as far as possible.	30°
	Lateral bending: Bend to the right, then left, as far as possible.	35° right to left
	Rotation: Twist upper trunk from the waist to the right, then to the left.	30° right to left

Shoulder	*Forward flexion:* Raise both arms forward and straight up over head.	180°
	Backward extension: Move both arms downward and back.	50°
	Abduction: Raise both arms laterally and straight up over head.	180° right and left
	Adduction: Move each arm across front of body.	50° right and left
	Internal rotation: Move both arms behind lower back with elbows out.	90°
	External rotation: Move both arms behind head with elbows out.	90°
Elbow	*Flexion:* Bend elbows, and touch hands to shoulders.	160° right and left
	Extension: Straighten elbows as much as possible.	0° right and left
	Supination: Bend elbows and hold against waist; rotate hands outward so palm is upward.	90° right and left
	Pronation: Elbows held as for supination; rotate hands inward so palms are downward.	90° right and left

*Deviations from these "normal" angles occur. The nurse should always compare one side of the body to the other when considering abnormal findings.

Continued

Table 16-4   Range of motion assessment—cont'd

Joint	Motion and Client Instructions	Measurement*
Wrist	*Flexion:* Bend both hands down at the wrist.	90° right and left
	Extension: Bend both hands up at the wrist.	70° right and left
	Ulnar deviation: Bend both wrists toward the little finger side of the hand.	55°
	Radial deviation: Bend both wrists toward the thumb side of the hand.	20°
Finger	*Flexion:* Make a tight fist.	Metacarpophalangeal: 90°
		Proximal phalangeal: 100°
		Distal phalangeal: 90°
	Extension: Open hand and extend fingers flat.	Metacarpophalangeal: 30°
		Proximal phalangeal joint: 0°
		Distal phalangeal joint: 20°
	Abduction: Spread fingers apart as far as possible.	20°
	Adduction: Close fingers together tightly.	0°
Thumb	*Flexion:* Move thumb over to base of little finger.	50°
	Extension: Move thumb away from rest of fingers.	0°
Hip	*Flexion:* Bend knees up to chest.	120°
	Extension: Lying prone, raise leg straight back.	20°

	Abduction: Move straight leg out to the side as far as possible.	45°
	Adduction: Bring legs back together, then cross one over the other.	30°
	Internal rotation: Flex knee and rotate leg inward toward other leg.	35°
	External rotation: Move outside of foot to opposite knee.	45°
Knee	*Flexion:* Bend each knee with calf touching thigh.	130°
	Extension: Straighten leg and stretch it.	15°
	Internal rotation: Move knee and lower leg inward.	10°
	External rotation: Move knee and lower leg outward.	10°
Ankle	*Dorsiflexion:* Point toes toward ceiling.	20°
	Plantar flexion: Point toes toward floor.	45°
	Inversion: Turn sole of foot toward middle.	30°
	Eversion: Turn sole of foot away from middle.	20°
Toe	*Flexion:* Curl toes under foot.	45°
	Extension: Raise toes upward.	70° to 90°

*Deviations from these "normal" angles occur. The nurse should always compare one side of the body to the other when considering abnormal findings.

Step	Normal/Individual Variations/Deviations
5. Maneuvers can be carried out in a variety of positions; select position based on client comfort and safety, with minimal changes required.	
6. Demonstrate maneuvers while instructing client.	
7. Be watchful of client for sudden loss of balance as maneuvers are performed; be prepared to provide support.	
8. Passive range of motion testing may be required if client is partially or fully immobilized.	
9. Use a goniometer only if gross joint motion reduction is suspected. Measure angles of greatest flexion and extension, and compare measurements with expected norms.	
Assess using the following special maneuvers if indicated: Straight leg-raising test (useful in determining herniated lumbar disk as cause of sciatic nerve pain)	Some tightness, but no pain. DEVIATIONS: Pain elicited before 70 degrees is reached; dorsiflexion aggravates the pain; pain relief with flexion of knee

Step	Normal/Individual Variations/Deviations
Technique: Have client lie on back on firm examination table with leg and thigh relaxed. Instruct to slowly raise foot while keeping knee straight, until pain elicited, then dorsiflex foot; repeat with other leg and compare.	
Ballottement (to determine the presence of excess fluid or an effusion in the knee)	No fluid wave or tap elicited. DEVIATIONS: Fluid wave or tap elicited
Technique: With client supine, knee extended, apply downward pressure on the suprapatellar pouch with the thumb and fingers of one hand, while pushing the patella sharply backward against the femur with a finger of the opposite hand. Quickly release the pressure against the patella while keeping the finger lightly touching the knee. A tap against the finger indicates an effusion.	
Bulge sign (to determine the presence of excess fluid in the knee)	No fluid wave or bulge on opposite side of joint DEVIATIONS: Fluid wave palpable on opposite side of joint

Step	Normal/Individual Variations/Deviations
Technique: With client supine and knee extended, milk medial aspect of knee upward two to three times; tap lateral side of patella. opposite side of joint	

Sample Documentation—Osteoporosis

Health History

Mrs. S., 67, reports she has been hearing a lot in the news lately about osteoporosis and is worried she may be at risk. States she is 1 inch shorter than she was in her twenties. Smokes ½ pack cigarettes/day for past 35 years. Denies alcohol use; drinks 2 cups coffee/day. Does not take calcium supplement, and eats/drinks very few foods/beverages with calcium. Denies fractures. Currently not taking any medications.

Physical Examination

Tall, thin; walks with smooth, regular rhythm and symmetric stride length; posture with increased dorsal kyphosis, and slight flexion of hips and knees; muscles and extremities symmetric. Muscle strength good overall, Grade 4. Active ROM in all joints without pain or gross limitation.

Client Teaching

Fall Prevention

1. Falls comprise the greatest number of accidents in older people. The causes of falls are numerous, but many falls are preventable. Normal, age-related changes that contribute to falls include altered posture and center of gravity, decreased reaction time, decreased muscle strength, and diminished vision. Chronic illness, medications, and environmental factors also contribute to the increased risk of falls.

2. Make modifications in your environment that are inexpensive and acceptable to you to reduce your own risk for a fall. Possibilities include the following:

   a. Use nonslip bath mats in tubs or showers.

   b. Place grab-bars at convenient locations near the tub and toilet for support.

   c. Use night lights to enable orientation to surroundings if you get up frequently at night.

   d. Use stable chairs with arms. Change positions slowly, and sit on side of bed for 1 minute before standing.

   e. Use rails for support and guidance on stairs.

   f. Since the need for light increases with age, increase the light in high-hazard areas such as stairs and stairwells.

   g. Check for and remove or stabilize common obstacles in your home like phone cords, extension cords, rugs, and carpet edges; place furniture and other objects out of traffic pathways.

3. Make a deliberate attempt to scan your environment as you walk to look for possible hazards.

4. Use mobility aids and assistive devices as prescribed.

5. Wear footwear with nonskid soles.

6. Develop an exercise program with your health care provider that includes aerobic conditioning, muscle strengthening, and gait or balance training.

References

Malasanos L et al: *Health assessment,* ed 4, St Louis, 1990, Mosby.

Thompson JM et al: *Mosby's clinical nursing,* ed 4, St Louis, 1997, Mosby.

Assessment of the Neurologic System

17

The central and peripheral components of the nervous system integrate all body functions. The neurologic system's function is to receive, store, process, and transmit information.

In the neurologic system assessment, the following are evaluated: mental and emotional status (refer to Chapter 5), cranial nerve function (integrated into previous chapters), motor and sensory function, and reflexes. The completeness and extent of assessment depend on the client's history and the purpose for which neurologic assessment is required. The minimum baseline assessment of the older client should include mental and emotional status, and motor and sensory function. Practice and judgment allow the examiner to make decisions about the extent of assessment.

Neurologic system assessment can be complicated by a variety of chronic disorders, as well as by normal, age-related changes. It may be necessary to perform this portion of the examination at a time separate from the remaining examination. Selected portions could also be performed over several sessions.

The skills of inspection, palpation, and percussion (with percussion or reflex hammer) are used. Equipment needs include sharp and dull testing implements, tuning fork (500 to 1000 cps), familiar objects (coin, paper clip), cotton wisp, and percussion hammer.

Anatomy and Physiology

The nervous system consists of two divisions: the central nervous system (brain and spinal cord) and the peripheral nervous system (cranial, spinal, and peripheral nerves). The peripheral nervous system is subdivided into the sensory, or afferent, division, and the motor, or efferent, division. The motor division, in turn, has two subdivisions: the somatic, or voluntary, nervous system, and the autonomic, or involuntary, nervous system. Sympathetic and para-sympathetic branches of the autonomic nervous system regulate nervous system activity.

The brain is composed of the cerebrum, cerebellum, and brain-stem (Fig. 17-1). The two cerebral hemispheres, each divided into lobes, comprise the greatest mass of the cerebrum. The outer layer, or cortex, integrates sensory and motor function and enables one

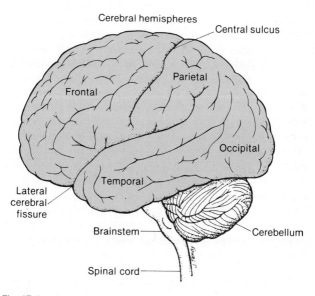

Fig. 17-1
The three major parts of the brain. (From Harkness G, Dincher J: *Medical-Surgical Nursing: total patient care*, ed 9, St Louis, 1996, Mosby.)

to carry out higher level functions that deal with behavior, learning, and language. The lobes of the brain are as follows:

Frontal: responsible for motor function and higher intellectual functions

Parietal: responsible for perception and integration of tactile sensations; also concerned with visual, gustatory, olfactory, and auditory sensations and proprioception

Temporal: responsible for the special senses of hearing, taste, and smell and for speech integration

Occipital: responsible for vision only

The cerebellum, like the cerebrum, is composed of an outer cortex and inner, white matter. The main functions of the cerebellum are maintaining balance, equilibrium, and muscular coordination.

The brainstem is the area through which all fibers pass to and from the spinal cord. It divides into the midbrain, pons, medulla oblongata, and diencephalon (Table 17-1 and Fig. 17-2).

The spinal cord extends from the foramen magnum to slightly above L2. The gray matter of the spinal cord is centrally located and surrounded by white matter. The gray matter is composed of nerve cell bodies, while the white matter consists of bundles of myelinated fibers containing sensory and motor neurons. Impulses are conducted through the ascending and descending tracts of the spinal cord within columns of white matter.

Twelve pairs of cranial nerves emerge from the various foramina of the skull. The first two pairs, olfactory and optic, emerge from the forebrain; the remaining emerge from the brainstem. All cranial nerves that have a motor function also have a sensory function. Some have both sensory and motor fibers, while others have only sensory or only motor fibers. Table 17-2 lists the name, number, and function of the cranial nerves.

The 31 pairs of spinal nerves are grouped as follows: eight cervical, twelve thoracic, five lumbar, five sacral, and one coccygeal. The nerves leave the spinal cord and vertebral canal through intervertebral foramina (Fig. 17-3). These nerves are mixed (sensory and motor) and are attached to the spinal cord by a dorsal (posterior) root composed of sensory fibers and a ventral (anterior) root composed of motor fibers. The sensory and motor fibers of each spinal nerve innervate the body dermatomes (Fig. 17-4, *A* and *B*).

A spinal nerve divides into several branches after emerging from the intervertebral foramen. A dorsal ramus branch innervates

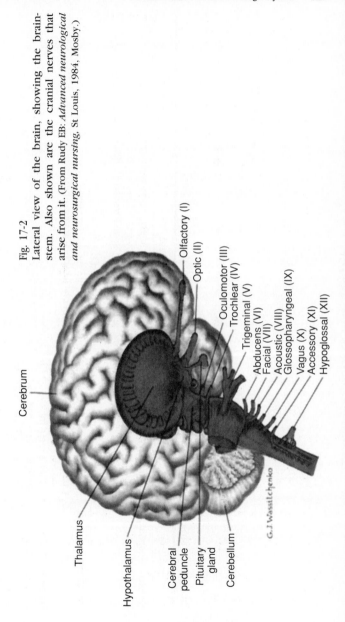

Fig. 17-2
Lateral view of the brain, showing the brain-stem. Also shown are the cranial nerves that arise from it. (From Rudy EB: *Advanced neurological and neurosurgical nursing*, St Louis, 1984, Mosby.)

Olfactory (I)
Optic (II)
Oculomotor (III)
Trochlear (IV)
Trigeminal (V)
Abducens (VI)
Facial (VII)
Acoustic (VIII)
Glossopharyngeal (IX)
Vagus (X)
Accessory (XI)
Hypoglossal (XII)

Cerebrum

Thalamus

Hypothalamus

Cerebral peduncle
Pituitary gland
Cerebellum

G.J Wassilchenko

Table 17-1   Structures of the brainstem and their functions, including the origin of cranial nerve (CN) nuclei

Structure	Function
Medulla oblongata CN IX-XII	Respiratory, circulatory, and vasomotor activities; houses respiratory center Reflexes of swallowing, coughing, vomiting, sneezing, and hiccupping Relay center for major ascending and descending spinal tracts that decussate at the pyramid
Pons CN V-VIII	Reflexes of pupillary action and eye movement Regulates respiration; houses a portion of the respiratory center Controls voluntary muscle action with corticospinal tract pathway
Midbrain CN III-IV	Reflex center for eye and head movement Auditory relay pathway Corticospinal tract pathway

Diencephalon CN I-II	
	Relays impulses between cerebrum, cerebellum, pons, and medulla
Thalamus	Conveys all sensory impulses (except olfaction) to and from cerebrum before their distribution to appropriate associative sensory areas
	Integrates impulses between motor cortex and cerebrum, influencing voluntary movements and motor response
	Controls state of consciousness, conscious perceptions of sensations, and abstract feelings
Epithalamus	Houses the pineal body
	Sexual development and behavior
Hypothalamus	Major processing center of internal stimuli for autonomic nervous system
	Maintains temperature control, water metabolism, body fluid osmolarity, feeding behavior, and neuroendocrine activity
Pituitary gland	Hormonal control of growth, lactation, vasoconstriction, and metabolism

From Seidel HM et al: *Mosby's guide to physical examination*, ed 3, St Louis, 1995, Mosby.

Table 17-2   Cranial nerves and their function

Cranial Nerves	Function
Olfactory (I)	Sensory: smell reception and interpretation
Optic (II)	Sensory: visual acuity and visual fields
Oculomotor (III)	Motor: raise eyelids, most extraocular movements
	Parasympathetic: pupillary constriction, change lens shape
Trochlear (IV)	Motor: downward, inward eye movement
Trigeminal (V)	Motor: jaw opening and clenching, chewing and mastication
	Sensory: sensation to cornea, iris, lacrimal glands, conjunctiva, eyelids, forehead, nose, nasal and mouth mucosa, teeth, tongue, ear, facial skin
Abducens (VI)	Motor: lateral eye movement

Facial (VII)	Motor: movement of facial expression muscles except jaw, closed eyes, labial speech sounds (*b*, *m*, *w*, and rounded vowels)
	Sensory: taste—anterior two thirds of tongue, sensation to pharynx
	Parasympathetic: secretion of saliva and tears
Acoustic (VIII)	Sensory: hearing and equilibrium
Glossopharyngeal (IX)	Motor: voluntary muscles for swallowing and phonation
	Sensory: sensation of nasopharynx, gag reflex, taste—posterior one third of tongue
	Parasympathetic: secretion of salivary glands, carotid reflex
Vagus (X)	Motor: voluntary muscles of phonation (guttural speech sounds) and swallowing
	Sensory: sensation behind ear and part of external ear canal
	Parasympathetic: secretion of digestive enzymes, peristalsis, carotid reflex, involuntary action of heart, lungs, and digestive tract
Spinal accessory (XI)	Motor: turn head, shrug shoulders, some actions for phonation
Hypoglossal (XII)	Motor: tongue movement for speech sound articulation (*l*, *t*, *n*) and swallowing

From Seidel HM et al: *Mosby's guide to physical examination*, ed 3, St Louis, 1995, Mosby.

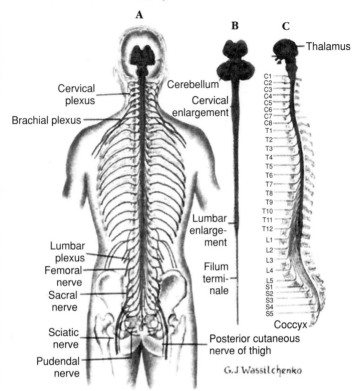

Fig. 17-3
Location of existing spinal nerves in relation to the vertebrae.
A, Posterior view, **B,** Anterior view of brainstem and spinal
cord. **C,** Lateral view of brainstem and spinal cord, showing relationship of spinal cord to vertebrae. (From Rudy EB: *Advanced
neurological and neurosurgical nursing,* St Louis, 1984, Mosby.)

the muscles, joints, and skin of the back along the vertebral column. A ventral ramus of a spinal nerve innervates the muscles and
skin of the lateral and ventral side of the torso. Except in the thoracic nerves T2 to T12, the ventral rami combine, then split again
as a network of nerves referred to as a plexus. The four plexuses
are cervical, brachial, lumbar, and sacral. Nerves emerge from the

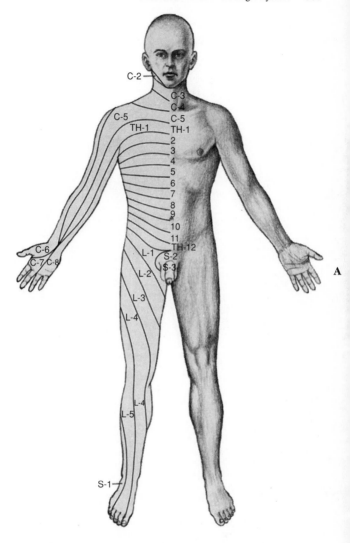

Fig. 17-4
A, Anterior view of sensory dermatomes. (**A** from Thompson JM et al: *Mosby's clinical nursing,* ed 3, St Louis, 1993, Mosby.)

Continued

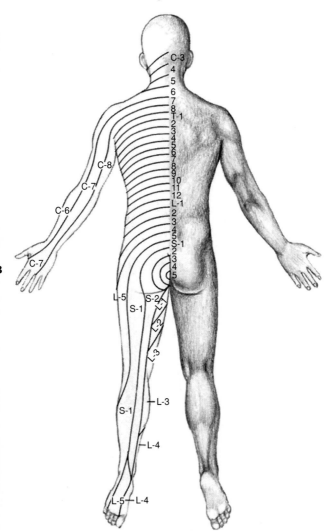

Fig. 17-4, cont'd
B, Posterior view of sensory dermatomes.

plexuses and are named according to the structures they innervate or general course taken (Fig. 17-3).

Nerve pathways provide routes for impulses traveling through the nervous system. The simplest type of nerve pathway is a reflex arc, the components of which are the receptor (in skin), sensory neuron, integration center (synapse[s]), motor neuron, and effector (usually skeletal muscle) (Fig. 17-5). The result of an impulse through a reflex arc is simply a reflex.

Common but inconsistently occurring structural age-related changes of the brain include atrophy of the gyri, widening of the sulci, and dilation of the ventricles. Neurons do not divide, so cell loss is permanent. An overall decrease in brain weight occurs. Demyelinization of nerve axons increases, and the number of axons decreases. Coupled with the decreased velocity of nerve impulse conduction, overall reaction time is delayed. Agility and fine motor coordination may be impaired. Benign essential tremor may appear with aging. Sense of touch and pain may be diminished. Deep tendon and superficial reflexes are present but may also be slightly decreased.

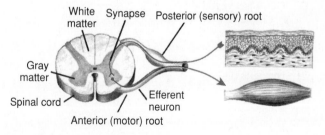

Fig. 17-5
Cross-section of the spinal cord showing a simple reflex arc.
(From Rudy EB: *Advanced neurological and neurosurgical nursing,* St Louis, 1984, Mosby.)

Assessment of the Neurologic System

Equipment needed:
Sharp and dull testing implements
Tuning fork (500 to 1000 cps)
Familiar objects (coin, paper clip)
Cotton wisp
Percussion hammer

Step	Normal/Individual Variations/Deviations
Cranial Nerves	
Examination described in other chapters:	
I Olfactory—Chapter 9	
II Optic—Chapter 8	
III Oculomotor—Chapter 8	
IV Trochlear—Chapter 8	
V Trigeminal (sensory)—Chapter 7	
Trigeminal (motor)—Chapter 7	
VI Abducens—Chapter 8	
VII Facial (sensory)—Chapter 9	
Facial (motor)—Chapter 7	
VIII Acoustic—Chapter 9	
IX Glossopharyngeal—Chapter 9	
X Vagus—Chapter 9	
XI Spinal accessory—Chapter 7	
XII Hypoglossal—Chapter 9	

Step	Normal/Individual Variations/Deviations

Proprioception and Cerebellar Function

Assess balance (NOTE: Use two of the following tests for gross screening.)

Gait

   Technique: Instruct client to walk barefoot for a short distance with eyes open, then turn and walk back with eyes closed. (CAUTION: Stand near client with your arms extended around, but not touching client, to prevent injury.) Note gait sequence, arm movements, and degree of steadiness.

   Continuous sequence of stance and arm swing with each step; smooth, regular rhythm with symmetric stride length, but may be slightly slower and more deliberate in movement; steps may be shortened with a widening distance between the feet

   DEVIATIONS: Gross unsteadiness, rigid or no arm movements; wide-based, shuffling, scissorslike, staggering, reeling, or parkinsonian gait

If abnormality identified in gait evaluation, instruct client to walk in tandem (heel-toe) fashion. Note exaggeration of any abnormality.

   Consistent contact between heel and toe; slight swaying

   DEVIATIONS: Instability with tendency to fall; steps to wider-base gait to maintain upright posture

Continued

Step	Normal/Individual Variations/Deviations
Equilibrium	Slight swaying (Romberg's sign negative)
Technique: Instruct client to stand erect, feet together, arms at sides with eyes open, then closed. (CAUTION: Stand nearby, prepared to intervene if client starts to fall.) Note degree of swaying. May also test equilibrium by instructing client to stand on one foot and then the other with eyes closed.	DEVIATIONS: Severe swaying or loss of balance Balance maintained for approximately 5 seconds with slight swaying (NOTE: Degree of musculoskeletal function will affect results and should be considered in evaluation.) DEVIATION: Unable to maintain balance
Assess coordination and proprioception:	
Rapid alternating movements	Smooth, rhythmic, purposeful, rapid-pace movement
Technique: Instruct client to pat knees with palms and backs of hands in rapid sequence.	DEVIATIONS: Clumsiness of movements and irregular timing
Finger-to-nose test	Smooth, rhythmic, accurate, rapid-paced movement
Technique: Instruct client to alternately touch finger to the nose with eyes open, then eyes closed; gradually increase speed.	DEVIATIONS: Clumsy movement; missed touch
Finger-to-finger test	Smooth, accurate, rapid-paced movement
Technique: Instruct client to touch finger to nose, then touch examiner's finger, which is 18 inches from client. Nurse then changes position of finger with increasing speed as client repeats the movement. Repeat with other hand.	DEVIATION: Unable to coordinate touch with examiner's finger

Step	Normal/Individual Variations/Deviations
Heel-to-shin test **Technique:** With client sitting, instruct to run heel of one foot up and down the opposite shin. Alternate with other heel and repeat maneuver several times.	Purposeful, accurate, smooth movement DEVIATIONS: Unable to coordinate movement; awkward or irregular movement
Sensory	
NOTE: The following tests should be performed on hands, lower arms, feet, and lower legs (facial sensation is described in Chapter 7). If impairment found, describe by the distribution of major peripheral nerves, or by dermatomes (see Fig. 17-4, *A* and *B*).	
Assess primary sensation: Light touch **Technique:** Lightly touch skin with a cotton wisp and instruct client to say "yes" when sensation is felt; client's eyes should be closed. Compare one side to the other.	Perception of light touch equal on both sides DEVIATIONS: Unable to perceive light touch, asymmetric response, or incorrect location identified

Continued

Step	Normal/Individual Variations/Deviations
Pain **Technique:** Touch skin in random fashion with sharp and dull instruments (e.g. point and hub of sterile needle). Instruct client to identify each touch as "sharp" or "dull"; client's eyes should be closed. Compare one side to the other.	Correct perception of pain equally on both sides DEVIATIONS: Unable to perceive pain; asymmetric response
Vibration **Technique:** Touch a vibrating tuning fork to bony prominences, beginning at the most distal joints (great toe, ankle, knee, finger, wrist, elbow may all be tested). Instruct client to say "yes" when vibration is first perceived and "now" when vibration stops. Damp the tines at different intervals to avoid consistency. Client's eyes should be closed. Compare one side to the other.	Accurate and equal perception of beginning and end of vibration at each bony prominence; occasionally decreased in fingers After age 70, decreased vibratory sense at ankle DEVIATIONS: Inaccurate or unequal perception of vibration at any bony prominence
Position **Technique:** Holding finger or toe joint in neutral position by the lateral aspects, raise or lower the digit. Instruct client to indicate "up" or "down." Client's eyes should be closed.	Accurate identification of position; may have decrease or absence of position in great toe DEVIATION: Incorrect identification of position

Step	Normal/Individual Variations/Deviations
Assess cortical and discriminatory sensation:	
Two-point discrimination **Technique:** Simultaneously touch selected body parts with two sharp objects. Instruct client to indicate if one or two points are felt; eyes should be closed.	Able to distinguish two points at the following minimal distances: Fingertips: 2-3 mm Palms: 8-12 mm Forearms: 40 mm Upper arms and thighs: 75 mm DEVIATION: Unable to distinguish two points within norms
Stereognosis **Technique:** Place familiar object in client's hand and instruct client to identify; eyes should be closed.	Correct identification DEVIATION: Incorrect identification
Graphesthesia **Technique:** Draw letter or number with blunt object on client's palm. Instruct client to identify figure; eyes should be closed.	Correct identification DEVIATION: Unable to distinguish
Point localization **Technique:** Touch an area on client's skin, then withdraw stimulus. Instruct client to identify spot touched.	Correct identification DEVIATION: Incorrect identification
Reflexes	
Assess superficial reflexes	(See Chapter 13, abdominal reflexes)
Assess deep tendon reflexes with percussion hammer (see box on pp. 344-345 and Table 17-3)	

Continued

Techniques and Strategies for Use of Percussion Hammer

1. The percussion hammer, like all other assessment tools, must be correctly used to obtain the desired response. Following are several strategies:
   a. The client must be relaxed and the extremities loose.
   b. The limb should be positioned so that there is slight tension on the tendon to be evaluated. For example, flex the knee to approximately 90 degrees before testing the patellar tendon.
   c. The examiner should hold the percussion hammer between the thumb and index finger loosely, so that as the examiner taps the desired tendon, the hammer is able to move smoothly and rapidly, yet in a controlled direction.
   d. The action of percussion with a hammer should be just like that of percussion used on the thorax or abdomen. The examiner should use a rapid wrist-flick motion to percuss the desired tendon. The tap should be quick, firm, and well directed. As soon as the tendon is tapped, the examiner should flick the wrist back so that the hammer does not remain on the tendon.
   e. Before the actual percussion, the examiner should palpate the desired tendon so that the precise location will be percussed.
2. If the client is heavy, deep tendon reflexes may be very difficult to elicit. The examiner should spend time trying to locate the tendon specifically before striking it with the hammer.

From Bowers AC, Thompson JM: *Clinical manual of health assessment,* ed 4, St Louis, 1992, Mosby.

Techniques and Strategies for Use of Percussion Hammer—cont'd

3. If the examiner has difficulty eliciting the deep tendon reflex in a client who shows no signs of neurologic dysfunction, several techniques may be tried.
   a. Change the client's position. If the client was sitting, try the technique with the client lying down. Any position may be used, as long as there is slight tension of the muscle or tendon being tested.
   b. If the examiner has difficulty eliciting the deep tendon reflex response of the lower extremity, it may be helpful to use the Jendrassik maneuver of reinforcement. The client locks the fingers together and pulls one hand against the other while the examiner attempts to elicit the lower leg reflexes.
   c. Reinforcement for the upper extremities may include instructing the client to tightly clench the teeth or tighten the muscles in the legs.
   d. If the examiner continues to have difficulty, the percussion technique should be reexamined.

Table 17-3   Scale of responses used to score deep tendon reflexes

Grade	Deep Tendon Reflex Response
0	No response
1+	Sluggish or diminished
2+	Active or expected response
3+	More brisk than expected, slightly hyperactive
4+	Brisk, hyperactive, with intermittent or transient clonus

From Seidel HM et al: *Mosby's guide to physical examination,* ed 3, St Louis, 1995, Mosby.

Step	Normal/Individual Variations/Deviations
Biceps **Technique:** Place client's forearm over your own opposite forearm, cupping client's elbow in your hand and placing thumb directly over tendon. Instruct client to completely relax arm, allowing you to support it. Strike your thumb with narrow end of hammer.	Visible or palpable flexion of forearms at elbow, bilaterally equal DEVIATIONS: Hyperactive or diminished response; asymmetric response
Brachioradialis **Technique:** Support client's arm in same manner as for biceps testing, but with client's hand slightly pronated. Strike radius with flat end of hammer, about 1 to 2 inches above wrist.	Flexion of elbow joint and pronation of forearm, bilaterally equal DEVIATIONS: As described above
Triceps **Technique:** Support client's arm in same manner as for biceps testing, but with elbow flexed to a greater degree (up to 90 degrees). Strike triceps tendon superior to the olecranon with narrow end of hammer.	Contraction of triceps muscle resulting in extension of arm at elbow, bilaterally equal DEVIATIONS: As described above

Step	Normal/Individual Variations/Deviations
Patellar	Contraction of quadriceps muscle resulting in extension of leg at knee; bilaterally equal
Technique: With client sitting on edge of examination table, legs dangling free, support upper leg with forearm or hand to keep it from resting against edge of table. Strike patellar tendon with flat end of hammer just below the patella.	DEVIATIONS: As described above
Ankle (Achilles)	Contraction of gastrocnemius muscle resulting in plantar flexion of foot, bilaterally equal; may be absent or difficult to elicit
Technique: With client sitting in same manner as for patellar, slightly dorsiflex the foot. Strike Achilles tendon with flat end of hammer at the level of the ankle malleoli.	DEVIATIONS: As described above
Assess pathologic reflexes	
Ankle clonus	No movement of foot
Technique: Support client's knee in partly flexed position while sharply dorsiflexing foot.	DEVIATIONS: Rhythmic oscillating movements between dorsiflexion and plantar flexion
Plantar (Babinski)	Flexion of toes; may be absent or difficult to elicit
Technique: Run handle of reflex hammer along lateral side of foot from heel to ball, then turn medially across ball toward great toe.	DEVIATIONS: Extension (dorsiflexion) of great toe with or without fanning of other toes

Sample Documentation—Alzheimer's Disease

Health History

Son of Mrs. W., 81, reports she has become increasingly more forgetful the past year, to the point that she is not able to pay her bills without his assistance; also having difficulty with cooking and eating. Mrs. W. claims she's not hungry, but he suspects she just doesn't remember to eat, since she has lost about 10 lb in the last 6 months. Mrs. W's granddaughter does her laundry for her, but Mrs. W. tends to wear the same clothes even though they are soiled.

Physical Examination

Alert, oriented to place and person. Quiet, reserved; does not initiate conversation. Hair uncombed, dirty. Nails ragged and dirty. Blouse soiled with food stains; strong body odor. Speech clear; able to follow simple instructions. Wanders off subject; some irrelevant responses. CN I-XII grossly intact. Wide-based, coordinated gait, but with shortened steps and stooped posture. Romberg negative. Rapid alternating movements slowed, but smooth and purposeful. Light touch, sharp/dull, and vibratory intact. DTRs 2+ bilaterally; plantar reflex negative. Short Blessed Test score 12/28.

References

Bowers AC, Thompson JM: *Clinical manual of health assessment,* ed 4, St Louis, 1992, Mosby.

Harkness G, Dincher J: *Medical-surgical nursing: total patient care,* ed 9, St Louis, 1996, Mosby.

Rudy EB: *Advanced neurological and neurosurgical nursing,* St Louis, 1984, Mosby.

Seidel HM et al: *Mosby's guide to physical examination,* ed 3, St Louis, 1995, Mosby.

Thompson JM et al: *Mosby's clinical nursing,* ed 3, St Louis, 1993, Mosby.

Appendix A
Sample Health History
and Physical Examination
Write-Up

Date: 5/18/97
Source and reliability of information: Self; reliable historian

1. **Client profile/biographical data**
   Bernice Nash
   2805 Spalding Drive
   St. Louis, MO 63116
   314-934-5644
   DOB: 1/19/20 Age: 77
   Widow, Caucasian, female
   Catholic
   Completed high school
   Contact person: Jeanne Emert (dau)
   3541 Evans Drive
   St. Louis, MO 63110
   314-840-1837

2. **Chief complaint/reason for visit**
   Here to establish care with new provider

3. **History of present problem**
   12 year h/o hypertension, well-controlled with diuretic; denies chest pain/pressure/heaviness, SOB/DOE/PND, headache, fatigue, lightheadedness. Last Chem 7 three mo ago— WNL. Taking medication as directed

4. **Family profile**

 Spouse: Jacob Nash, Deceased, 1979, throat cancer

 Children: daughter Jeanne Emert (see above)

5. **Occupational profile**

 Retired teacher

 Income sources: Social Security, teacher's pension, investment income; states adequate for needs

6. **Living environment profile**

 3-bedroom ranch-style home, well-maintained, with LR, DR, kitchen, 2 bathrooms, basement; lives alone; neighbors on both sides whom she sees/interacts with regularly

7. **Recreation/leisure profile**

 Enjoys bird watching, walking, needlepoint, gardening; docent at area zoo

 Member of church women's club

 Travels yearly to Georgia to visit sister for 2 weeks; takes about 6 additional day trips a year with women's club

8. **Resources/support systems used**

 Physician: Dr. Ellen MacPeek, 4600 Chippewa, St. Louis, MO 63116

 Hospital: St. John's

 No other health care resources/agencies involved

9. **Description of typical day**

 Awakens at 7 AM, reads newspaper while eating breakfast. Usually cleans house, does laundry, or gardens in mornings. Eats lunch about noon, 2-3 times a week goes out with friends. Does needlework in afternoons while watching soap operas for 2 hours, or works in gardens around her home. Dinner about 5:30 PM, usually alone. Reads, watches TV in evenings. To bed after 10 PM news. Spends 1 day a week at zoo doing volunteer work, occasionally more.

10. **Present health status**

 No health problems this past year

 Had cholecystectomy 2 years ago (1995); occasional pain and stiffness in hands with needlework, and in hips and knees with gardening; diagnosed with hypertension 4 years ago (1993)

 Worried that arthritis will gradually get worse and severely limit her activities

Requires no special treatments/therapies

Remains functional within the constraints of above noted symptoms; takes ibuprofen 200 mg tablets 2 every 4-6 hr prn, usually about twice a day

Medications

HCTZ 50 mg daily with orange juice, Dr. MacPeek, 4/22/97

Ibuprofen as noted above

Centrum Silver multivitamin 1 daily

Denies side effects of meds; ibuprofen provides adequate relief; no difficulty obtaining meds; affordable

Immunization status

Tetanus: 1989

PPD: 1990

Influenza: fall, 1996

Pneumovax: never

Allergies

Sulfa results in full body rash; denies food, substance, or seasonal allergies

Nutrition

24-hour diet recall:

Breakfast at 7 AM—2 cups of coffee, 6 oz orange juice, shredded wheat with fresh strawberries and 2% milk, 1 scrambled egg substitute

Lunch at noon—out with friends; chicken salad sandwich on croissant, small bowl of fresh fruit salad, iced tea

Dinner at 5:30—broiled hamburger patty on bun with lettuce and tomato, mustard, $\frac{1}{2}$ baked potato, $\frac{1}{2}$ cup green beans, 1 cup coffee

Drinks four 8 oz glasses of water daily

Tries to limit salt intake by not cooking with salt or adding it at the table; likes fresh fruits and vegetables

Weight stable at 140 lb the past 15 years

Denies problems with purchasing or preparing foods

11. **Past health status**

Childhood illnesses

Exact illnesses or dates unknown, but recalls having measles, mumps, chickenpox

Serious or chronic illnesses

1993—hypertension

1980—osteoarthritis (generalized)

Trauma

1955—auto accident; fx. right-sided ribs

1972—fell on ice and sustained fx. fibula; casted

Hospitalizations

1948, City Hospital—delivery of first child, Dr. Glaser

1955, City Hospital—rib fractures, Dr. Becker

1995, St. John's—cholecystectomy, Dr. James

Obstetric history

$G_1P_1A_0$

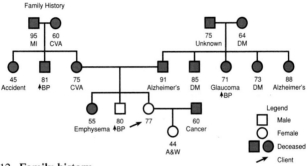

Family History

Legend

☐ Male
◯ Female
■ ● Deceased
↗ Client

12. **Family history**

13. **Review of systems**

General

Increased fatigue with spring and fall gardening activities; denies weight change, appetite change, fever, night sweats, difficulty sleeping, frequent colds/infections; rates overall health as "very good"; manages all ADLs and IADLs independently.

Integument

Multiple "red moles" on chest and abdomen, and multiple flat, brown moles throughout body, but no other lesions; denies pigment changes. Denies pruritus, hair or nail changes/problems.

Hematopoietic

Bruises easily. No h/o anemia. Has never had blood transfusion.

Head

Occasional mild frontal headache with too much needlework; no associated symptoms, and relieved by 2 acetaminophen tablets. Denies h/o trauma, dizziness.

Eyes

Wears trifocal glasses since about age 48; no recent vision changes noted; denies pain, tearing, pruritus, swelling, floaters, diplopia, blurring, photophobia; last eye exam 11/96, and sees optometrist annually.

Ears

Denies hearing loss, discharge, pain, tinnitus; no h/o infections. Audiometric screening done 1995. Washes ears daily with washcloth only.

Nose and sinuses

Denies rhinorrhea, discharge, epistaxis, obstruction; denies sinus pain, postnasal drip, or allergies. Rare sinus infection, last one about 5 years ago. Olfactory sensation intact.

Mouth and throat

Denies sore throats, hoarseness or voice change, difficulty swallowing; occasional "fever blister" on right upper lip, usually when exposed to too much sun in summer; treats with Blistex OTC salve and gets relief; no difficulty eating/chewing food and taste is intact; no dental appliances; sees dentist every 6 mo; brushes twice daily and flosses once daily.

Neck

Denies pain, stiffness, limited ROM, or masses.

Breasts

Denies lumps/masses, pain/tenderness, nipple discharge or changes; does not perform BSE and has never had a mammogram.

Respiratory

Denies cough, dyspnea, hemoptysis, wheezing; does not recall having a CXR.

Cardiovascular

Denies chest pain/discomfort, palpitations, SOB/DOE/PND, or orthopnea; noted BLE edema before being diagnosed with high blood pressure, but only gets it now in the summer with high temperatures; no varicosities, claudication, paresthesias, or color changes in extremities; no known heart murmur.

Gastrointestinal

Denies dysphagia, indigestion, n/v, hematemesis, pain, food intolerances, or appetite change; no diarrhea, constipation, melena, rectal bleeding; had hemorrhoids with pregnancy,

but not recurrence; has soft, brown stool daily after breakfast. Denies jaundice.

Urinary

Denies dysuria, frequency, dribbling, hesitancy, hematuria,
polyuria; notes occasional incontinence with coughing,
sneezing, and laughing for which she wears a panty liner;
no nocturia, h/o stones or infection. Urine clear, light
yellow.

Genitoreproductive

Denies lesions, discharge, pain, itching. Sexually inactive. No
h/o STDs. Onset of menarche at age 13; LMP at age 53; no
use of HRT. Last PAP smear 1996—WNL.

Musculoskeletal

Fingers, knees, and hips with periodic pain and stiffness,
usually worse on arising, relieved by 2 ibuprofen tablets
after about an hour; no heat, redness, swelling of these
same joints, and no effect on ADLs; denies muscle
weakness, gait problems, back pain. Walks daily during
good weather about 15-20 minutes; no other formal
exercise program.

Central nervous system

Denies syncopal attacks, LOC, seizures, paralysis/paresis, balance or coordination problems, paresthesias, tics/tremors,
or h/o head injury; denies memory problems.

Endocrine system

Denies heat/cold intolerance, h/o goiter, skin/hair changes,
polyphagia, polydipsia, or polyuria.

Psychosocial

Denies depression, stating "my life is full and rewarding,"
though admits to feeling occasionally anxious about getting
older and the effect it will have on her independence. Denies insomnia, nervousness, fear; no trouble with decision
making or concentration. Describes self as "satisfied" and
denies difficulty coping with daily stresses.

Physical Examination

General

77-year-old white female, appearing stated age; alert, well
groomed, articulate; makes eye contact and responds appropriately to questions.

T98° F, P68, R16, BP140/82 sitting R arm

Wt. 141 lb, Ht. 5'6"

Skin

Light color, even throughout, well-lubricated; turgor with delayed recoil; multiple scattered cherry angiomas on trunk, ranging in size from 2-5 mm; no other lesions noted; nail beds pink without clubbing; hair with coarse texture, thinning and gray, female distribution.

Head

Normocephalic. Scalp pink, without lesions or tenderness; symmetric facial features.

Eyes

Distant vision with glasses 20/30 OU; near vision 20/20 OU with glasses.

Visual fields normal by confrontation; EOMs normal, without nystagmus. Lashes and brows evenly distributed, with thin brows; lids symmetric with slight upper lid ptosis OU; equal palpebral fissure height. Conjunctivae clear, sclerae white. Corneas with arcus senilis present. Anterior chamber slightly shallow but transparent. Iris blue, round bilaterally. PERRLA. Lens clear. Red reflex present but with early gray-green cataracts present, R>L. Fundi normal without AV nicking, hemorrhages, or exudates.

Ears

Auricles aligned symmetrically, without lesions, nodules, or tenderness. Canals with small amount of dark amber, soft cerumen AU; TMs pearly gray, translucent, with landmarks and light reflex present; no perforations. Watch tick heard AU at 2 inches. Weber: no lateralization. Rinne: AC 2 × >BC.

Nose and sinuses

No nasal flaring; nares patent; identified coffee and cloves. Mucosa pink, moist, without discharge; septum intact without deviation or perforation; turbinates without swelling, polyps, or lesions. No frontal or maxillary sinus tenderness.

Mouth and throat

Buccal mucosa pink, moist, and without lesions. Teeth in excellent repair; gums pink with tight margins. Tongue pink, smooth, moist without lesions. Tongue protrudes in midline, symmetric movement. Uvula in midline on phonation, gag reflex intact; pharynx pink, without exudate. Differentiates sweet and sour tastes.

Neck

Full ROM, veins not distended. Carotid pulsations equal and of good quality. Trachea in midline. Thyroid not palpable. No lymphadenopathy.

Breasts

Symmetric, with R slightly larger than L; large, pendulous, and flabby; smooth texture. No masses or tenderness, no retraction or discharge. No lymphadenopathy.

Chest and lungs

Thorax symmetric, expansion equal bilaterally. AP diameter not increased. Tactile fremitus equal bilaterally; lung fields resonant throughout; diaphragmatic excursion 4 cm bilaterally. Breath sounds CTA anterior, posterior, and lateral.

Heart and blood vessels

No heave or lift; apical impulse at 5th LICS just medial to MCL. RRR, S_1 and S_2 without splitting, with grade II/VI SEM heard in all areas; no gallop, rubs.

JVP visible at sternal angle with 40-degree elevation. Peripheral pulses 2+ throughout bilaterally. No carotid or abdominal bruits. BLE without edema, tenderness; warm, pink.

Abdomen

Rounded, protuberant with few silvery white striae over lower abdomen; symmetric, without bulging; 12 cm healed scar RUQ (cholecystectomy). BS present all 4 quadrants. No masses or tenderness on palpation; spleen, kidneys nonpalpable; liver edge at costal margin nontender; liver 11 cm percussed dullness.

Musculoskeletal

Arms and legs symmetric with overall general appearance of flexion; muscles appear symmetric with good strength, equal bilaterally; full active and passive ROM; no tenderness, swelling, heat, or erythema noted. Slight kyphosis.

Neurologic

Alert and oriented × 3; relates history in clear, logical manner with some reminiscence noted; recent and remote memory intact with SBT score of 2/28; mood appropriate to subject discussed. CNs I-XII grossly intact. Finger-to-nose, heel-to-shin smooth and purposeful. Light touch, sharp/dull, and vibratory intact and equal bilaterally. Gait normal, Romberg negative.

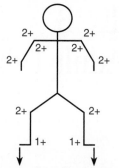

Deep tendon reflex response

Genitoreproductive
Thin, sparse, gray, straight pubic hair in female distribution
pattern. BUS: no tenderness, erythema, or discharge. Labia
symmetric, pale pink, dry. Introitus small without pro-
lapses. Vagina pale pink, no rugae, slightly moist; cervix
centrally placed; no discharge. Uterus and adnexae nonpalpable. Slightly lax anal sphincter tone; no hemorrhoids or
masses noted; smooth rectal walls; soft brown stool guaiac
negative.

Appendix B
Older Adult Laboratory Values

Test	General Trend from Standards	Range
Hematology		
Hemoglobin	Decreases to lower limits of normal	M—12.4-14.9 g/100 ml F—11.7-13.8 g/100 ml Lower standard ranges
Hematocrit	Decreases to lower limits of normal	M—42%-54% F—38%-46% Lower limits of standard range
Sedimentation rate	Mild increase	0-20 units
Chemistry		
Albumin	Decreases slightly	3.3-4.9 g/100 ml
Creatinine	Increases	0.6-1.8 mg/100 ml*
BUN	Increases	M—8-35 mg/100 ml F—6-30 mg/100 ml
Potassium	Increases slightly	Runs higher to upper limits of standard
Glucose	Increases somewhat	150 mg/100 ml proposed upper limit†

Data compiled from Andresen (1989) and Jeppesen (1986) in Hogstel MO: *Clinical manual of gerontological nursing,* St Louis, 1992, Mosby, and Tripp TR: Laboratory and diagnostic tests. In Lueckenotte AG: *Textbook of gerontologic nursing,* St. Louis, 1996, Mosby.

*Age and creatinine must be taken into account; may have normal values even in renal failure.

†Common to have higher values but reflects carbohydrate intolerance.

Test	General Trend from Standards	Range
Chemistry—cont'd		
Calcium	Decreases slightly	8.2-10.5 mg/100 ml
Uric acid	Increases some-what	7.7 mg/100 ml upper limit of standard
Enzymes		
Alkaline phos-phatase	Increases slightly	M—80 units average F—79 units average
Urine chemistry		
Creatinine clear-ance	Must be calculated for age-related changes*	
Specific gravity	Decreases maximum value	1.028-1.024
Blood gases		
P_{CO_2}	Increases slightly	35-45 mm Hg
P_{O_2}	Decreases	80-100 mm Hg
Hormones		
Thyroid stimula-tion hormone (TSH)	Increases†	0.4-4.9 UIU/ml

*Creatinine clearance calculated as $\dfrac{(140 - \text{age}) \times \text{Body weight (kg)}}{\text{Serum creatinine} \times 72 \text{ kg}}$
($\times$ 0.85 for women)
†Common but related to abnormal thyroid function.

Appendix C
Managing Acute
and Chronic Urinary
Incontinence

Purpose and Scope

Urinary incontinence (UI) affects approximately 13 million Americans or about 10-35 percent of adults and at least half of the 1.5 million nursing home residents. Among the population between 15 and 64 years of age, the prevalence of UI in men ranges from 1.5 to 5 percent and in women from 10 to 30 percent. For noninstitutionalized persons older than 60 years of age, prevalence ranges from 15 to 35 percent, with women having twice the prevalence of men. Survey data from caregivers of the elderly show that approximately 53 percent of the homebound elderly are incontinent. A random sampling of hospitalized elderly patients identified 11 percent as having persistent UI at admission and 23 percent at discharge. A recent estimate of the direct costs of caring for persons of all ages with incontinence is more than $15 billion annu-

Fantl JA, Newman DK, Colling J, et al. *Managing Acute and Chronic Urinary Incontinence.* Clinical Practice Guideline. Quick Reference Guide for Clinicians, No. 2, 1996 Update. Rockville, MD: U.S. Department of Health and Human Services, Public Health Service, Agency for Health Care Policy and Research. AHCPR Pub. No. 96-0686. March 1996.

Abbreviations used in this guideline: **BUN** Blood urea nitrogen; **DHIC** Detrusor hyperactivity with impaired bladder contractility; **DI** Detrusor instability; **ISD** Intrinsic sphincter deficiency; **NSAID** Nonsteroidal anti-inflammatory drug; **PME** Pelvic muscle exercise; **PPA** Phenylpropanolamine; **PVR** Postvoid residual volume; **SUI** Stress urinary incontinence; **TCA** Tricyclic antidepressant; **UI** Urinary incontinence; **UTI** Urinary tract infection.

ally. Despite the high prevalence and considerable cost burden of the condition, most affected individuals do not seek help for incontinence. Studies indicate, however, that treatment is effective in most people with UI.

UI is defined as involuntary loss of urine that is sufficient to be a problem. UI can be caused by factors affecting either the anatomy or the physiology of the lower urinary tract, or both, as well as other factors. The symptoms and subtypes of UI are outlined in Table C-1. Documented risk factors associated with incontinence are wide-ranging and include:

- Immobility commonly associated with chronic degenerative disease.
- Diminished cognitive status and delirium.
- Medications, including diuretics.
- Smoking.
- Fecal impaction.
- Low fluid intake.
- Environmental barriers.
- High-impact physical activities.
- Diabetes.
- Stroke.
- Estrogen depletion.
- Pelvic muscle weakness.
- Pregnancy, vaginal delivery, and episiotomy.

Specific risk factors for incontinence can be both identified and remediated with targeted intervention. Examples of possible preventive maneuvers include teaching women about gestational and postpartum pelvic muscle exercises, and teaching both men and women about scheduled voiding and proper bladder-emptying techniques. Other health promotion models describe education programs regarding estrogen use to treat atrophic vaginitis, postmenopausal changes of the genitourinary tract, and elimination of fluids with diuretic effects.

The findings and recommendations included in the *Clinical Practice Guideline Update* define a comprehensive program for managing UI in adults. This *Quick Reference Guide* is intended for health care providers who examine and treat adults with this condition. The guide does not address involuntary loss of urine through channels other than the urethra (extraurethral UI), UI in children, or UI due to neuropathic conditions.

Table C-1   Symptoms and subtypes of urinary incontinence

Type of UI	Definition	Pathophysiology	Symptoms and Signs
Urge	Involuntary loss of urine associated with a strong sensation of urinary urgency	■ Involuntary detrusor (bladder) contractions (detrusor instability (DI)). ■ Detrusor hyperactivity with impaired bladder contractility (DHIC).	Loss of urine with an abrupt and strong desire to void; usually loss of urine on way to bathroom. DHIC—elevated post-void residual (PVR) volume.
		■ Involuntary sphincter relaxation.	Involuntary loss of urine (without symptoms).
Stress	Urethral sphincter failure usually associated with increased intra-abdominal pressure	■ Urethral hypermobility due to anatomic changes or defects such as fascial detachments (hypermobility).	Small amount of urine loss during coughing, sneezing, laughing, or other physical activities.
		■ Intrinsic urethral sphincter deficiency (ISD) failure of the sphincter at rest.	Continuous leak at rest or with minimal exertion (postural changes).
Mixed	Combination of urge and stress UI	■ Combination of urge and stress UI features as above. ■ Common in women, especially older women.	Combinations of urge and stress UI symptoms as above. One symptom (urge or stress) often more bothersome to the patient than the other.
Overflow	Bladder overdistention	■ Acontractile detrusor. ■ Hypotonic or underactive detrusor secondary to drugs, fecal impaction, diabetes, lower spinal cord injury, or disruption of the motor innervation of the detrusor muscle. ■ In men—secondary obstruction due to prostatic hyperplasia, prostatic carcinoma, or urethral stricture.	Variety of symptoms, including frequent or constant dribbling or urge or stress incontinence symptoms, as well as urgency and frequent urination.

Table C-1   Symptoms and subtypes of urinary incontinence—cont'd

Type of UI	Definition	Pathophysiology	Symptoms and Signs
		■ In women—obstruction due to severe genital prolapse or surgical overcorrection of urethral detachment.	
Other			
Functional	Chronic impairments of physical and/or cognitive functioning	■ Chronic functional and mental disabilities.	Urge incontinence or functional limitations.
Unconscious or reflex	Neurologic dysfunction	■ Decreased bladder compliance with risk of vesicoureteral reflux and hydronephrosis. ■ Secondary to radiation cystitis, inflammatory bladder conditions, radical pelvic surgery, or myelomenigocele. ■ In many nonneurogenic cases, no demonstrable DI.	Postmicturitional or continual incontinence. Severe urgency with bladder hypersensitivity (sensory urgency).

Highlights of Patient Management

Effective management of UI in primary care should focus on:

- Assessment of the patient and the incontinence.
- Identification of risk factors and reversible causative conditions.
- Treatment of reversible conditions.
- Discussion of UI treatment options.
- Implementation of an effective plan of management consistent with the patient's condition, goals, and wishes.
- Education and quality-of-life improvement.

Figure C-1 is an overview of the evaluation and management of UI in primary care and displays the decision points and preferred management pathways outlined in this guide.

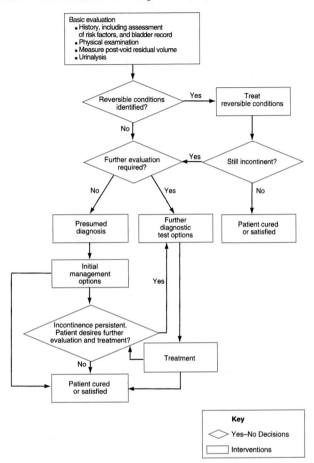

Fig. C-1
Evaluation and management of urinary incontinence in primary care.

Incontinence Profile

Questions such as those listed below are useful in the initial identification and assessment of UI.

- Can you tell me about the problems you are having with your bladder?

OR

- Can you tell me about the trouble you are having holding your urine (water)?
- How often do you lose urine when you don't want to?
- When do you lose urine when you don't want to? What activities or situations are linked with leakage? Is it associated with laughing, coughing, or getting to the bathroom?
- How often do you wear a pad for protection?
- Do you use other protective devices to collect your urine?
- How long have you been having a problem with urine leakage?

Basic Evaluation Checklist

History

The history should include a focused medical, neurologic, and genitourinary history that includes an assessment of risk factors, a review of medications, and a detailed exploration of the symptoms of the UI and associated symptoms and factors, including the following:

- Duration and characteristics of UI (see Incontinence Profile).
- Most bothersome symptom(s) to the patient.
- Frequency, timing, and amount of continent voids and incontinent episodes.
- Precipitants of incontinence (e.g., situational antecedents, such as cough, laugh, or exercises "on way to bathroom"; surgery; injury/trauma; recent illness; new medications).
- Other urinary tract symptoms (e.g., nocturia, dysuria, hesitancy, enuresis, straining, poor or interrupted stream, pain).
- Daily fluid intake.
- Bowel habits.
- Alteration in sexual function due to UI.
- Amount and type of perineal pads or protective devices.
- Previous treatments and effects on UI.
- Expectations of treatment.

Mental Status Evaluation

- Cognition.
- Motivation to self toilet.

Functional Assessment

- Manual dexterity.
- Mobility
  ○ Observe patient toileting.
  ○ Can patient toilet unaided?
  ○ Are physical or chemical restraints being used?

Environmental Assessment

- Access and distance to toilets or toilet substitutes.
- Chair/bed allows ease when rising.

Social Factors

- Relationship of UI to work.
- Living arrangements.
- Identified caregiver and degree of caregiver involvement.
- Lives alone.

Bladder Records

See Figure C-2.
- Frequency, timing, and amount of voids.
- Amount of incontinent episodes.
- Activities associated with UI.
- Fluid intake.

Physical Examination

Guided by the medical history, the physical examination includes:
- General examination
  ○ Edema.
  ○ Neurologic abnormalities.
- Abdominal examination
  ○ Diastasis rectii (separation of the rectus muscles of the abdominal wall).
  ○ Organomegaly.
  ○ Masses.
  ○ Peritoneal irritation.
  ○ Fluid collections.

NAME: _____

DATE: _____

INSTRUCTIONS: Place a check in the appropriate column next to the time you urinated in the toilet or when an incontinence episode occurred. Note the reason for the incontinence and describe your liquid intake (for example, coffee, water) and estimate the amount (for example, one cup).

Time interval	Urinated in toilet	Had a small incontinence episode	Had a large incontinence episode	Reason for incontinence episode	Type/amount of liquid intake
6–8 a.m.					
8–10 a.m.					
10–noon					
Noon–2 p.m.					
2–4 p.m.					
4–6 p.m.					
6–8 p.m.					
8–10 p.m.					
10–midnight					
Overnight					

No. of pads used today: _____ No. of episodes: _____

Comments: _____

_____

_____

Fig. C-2
Sample bladder record.

- Rectal examination
  - Perineal sensation.
  - Resting and active sphincter tone.
  - Fecal impaction.
  - Masses.
  - Consistency and contour of the prostate (men).

- Genital examination in men
  - Skin condition.
  - Abnormalities of the foreskin, penis, and perineum.
- Pelvic examination in women
  - Skin condition.
  - Genital atrophy.
  - Pelvic organ prolapse.
  - Pelvic masses.
  - Perivaginal muscle tone.
  - Other abnormalities.
- Direct observation of urine loss
  - Urine loss with full bladder using cough stress test.
- Estimation of post-void residual (PVR) volume.
- Urinalysis.

Supplementary Assessments

Supplementary assessments may be necessary or helpful in some patients, including:
- Blood testing (BUN, creatinine, calcium)
  - Suspected compromised renal function.
  - Polyuria.

Initial Care

After the basic evaluation, treatment for the presumed type of UI (see Table C-1) should be initiated unless further evaluation by a specialist is indicated. All incontinent patients with identified reversible conditions that cause or contribute to UI should be managed appropriately. Table C-2 lists reversible conditions and their management.

Further Evaluation

Patients requiring further evaluation include those who meet any of the criteria listed in Table C-3.

Please note that specialized testing, including urodynamic, endoscopic, and imaging tests, is not detailed here. Although primary health care providers are not expected to be experts in these techniques, they should be familiar with the diagnostic test options for evaluating the symptoms of UI. The tests are performed by qualified professionals trained in the specific definitions and proce-

Table C-2   Identification and management of reversible conditions that cause or contribute to urinary incontinence

Condition	Comment	Management
Conditions Affecting the Lower Urinary Tract		
Urinary tract infection	Dysuria and urgency from symptomatic infection may defeat the older person's ability to reach the toilet in time, causing urge incontinence. Asymptomatic infection, although more common than symptomatic infection, is rarely a cause of incontinence.	Treat symptomatic urinary tract infection (UTI) with antibiotics.
Atrophic urethritis or vaginitis	Hypoestrogenism causes atrophic changes of the lower genitourinary tract. Although its association to incontinence and sensory symptoms has long been suspected, direct cause–effect has not yet been proven.	Estrogen replacement therapy
Pregnancy/vaginal delivery/episiotomy	Pelvic floor anatomic and physiologic changes (e.g., fetal pressure, hormonal changes) may temporarily alter continence physiology	Behavioral intervention. Condition may be self-limiting. Conservative management recommended.
Postprostatectomy	Disruption of sphincter mechanisms may or may not be permanent.	Behavioral intervention. Avoid surgical therapy until clear condition will not resolve.
Stool impaction	Patients with stool impaction present with either urge or overflow incontinence. Stool impaction may induce fecal incontinence as well.	Disimpaction restores continence in most instances if this was the cause. Implement a bowel regimen: appropriate use of stool softeners, bulk-forming agents, and laxatives if necessary; implement high fiber intake, adequate mobility, and fluid intake.

Continued

Table C-2   Identification and management of reversible conditions that cause or contribute to urinary incontinence—cont'd

Condition	Comment	Management
Drug Side Effects*		
Diuretics	The brisk diuresis induced by diuretics may precipitate incontinence. This is particularly relevant in older persons and in those in whom continence is already impaired. Diuretics were observed to increase the severity of UI in already incontinent persons.	Discontinue or change therapy if clinically possible. Changing time of administration of diuretic may alter incontinence.
Caffeine	Diuretic effect may aggravate or precipitate UI.	Eliminate caffeine intake or substitute with decaffeinated products.
Anticholinergic agents Psychotropics Antidepressants (TCAs) Phenothiazines Disopyramide Antispasmodics Anti-parkinsonian agents	Prescription as well as over-the-counter drugs with anticholinergic properties are taken commonly by patients with insomnia, coryza, pruritus, vertigo, and other symptoms or conditions. Anticholinergic side effects include urinary retention with associated urinary frequency and overflow incontinence. In addition to anticholinergic actions, antipsychotics such as thorazine and haloperidol may cause sedation, rigidity, and immobility.	Discontinue use if clinically appropriate.
Narcotic analgesics Sedatives/ hypnotics/CNS depressants/ alcohol	Benzodiazepines, especially long-acting agents such as flurazepam and diazepam, may accumulate in elderly patients and cause confusion and secondary incontinence. Diazepam can have a strong anticholinergic effect. Alcohol, frequently used as a sedative, can cloud the sensorium, impair mobility, and induce a diuresis, resulting in incontinence.	Discontinue use if clinically possible.

*Many side effects are seen with over-the-counter drugs, the use of which may not be reported by some patients.

Table C-2   Identification and management of reversible conditions that cause or contribute to urinary incontinence—cont'd

Condition	Comment	Management
Alpha-adrenergic agents Antihistamines Sympathomimetics (decongestants) Sympatholytics (e.g., prazosin, terazosin, and doxazosin) Beta-adrenergic agonists	Alpha-adrenergic stimulation increases urethral tone and alpha-adrenergic block reduces it. Alpha-agonists may induce retention symptoms in older men. Stress incontinence may become symptomatic in a woman treated with alpha-antagonist as antihypertensive therapy. An older man with prostate enlargement or a woman with severe genital prolapse may develop acute urinary retention and overflow incontinence when taking multicomponent "cold" capsules that contain alpha-agonists and anticholinergic agents, especially if a nasal decongestant and a nonprescription hypnotic antihistamine are added.	Discontinue use if clinically appropriate.
Calcium channel blockers	Calcium channel blockers can reduce smooth muscle contractility in the bladder and occasionally can cause urinary retention and overflow incontinence.	Discontinue use if clinically appropriate.
Increased Urine Production		
Metabolic (hyperglycemia, hypercalcemia) Excess fluid intake Volume overload Venous insufficiency with edema Congestive heart failure	Excess intake, endocrine conditions that cloud the sensorium and induce a diuresis (e.g., hypercalcemia, hyperglycemia, and diabetes insipidus), and expanded volume states such as congestive heart failure, lower extremity venous insufficiency, drug-induced ankle edema (e.g., nifedipine, indomethacin), and low albumin states can cause polyuria and can lead to incontinence by unduly rapid and excessive filling of the bladder.	Treatment of the underlying condition. Implement bladder retraining to assist with frequency.

Continued

Table C-2   Identification and management of reversible conditions that cause or contribute to urinary incontinence—cont'd

Condition	Comment	Management
Impaired Ability or Willingness to Reach a Toilet		
Delirium	In the delirious patient, incontinence is usually an associated symptom that will abate with proper diagnosis and treatment of the underlying cause of confusion.	Reassess patient for possible bladder retraining once delirium abates.
Psychological	The relationship between psychological conditions and UI is still poorly understood as cause–effect are still controversial.	Treatment of the psychological disorder.
Restricted mobility	Limited mobility is an aggravating or precipitating cause of incontinence that can frequently be corrected or improved by treating the underlying chronic illness or injury (e.g., arthritis, poor eyesight, Parkinson's disease, or orthostatic hypotension). A urinal or bedside commode and scheduled toileting often help resolve the incontinence that results from hospitalization and its environmental barriers (e.g., bed rails, restraints, and poor lighting).	Treatment of underlying condition, facilitation of toileting facilities, and use of toileting aids and devices.

dures. The specialized diagnostic tests are reviewed in the *Clinical Practice Guideline Update.*

Treatment Options

The three major categories of treatment are behavioral, pharmacologic, and surgical. Treatment options, including their risks, benefits, and outcomes, should be discussed with the patient so that informed choices can be made. As a general rule, the first choice should be the least invasive treatment with the fewest potential adverse effects that is appropriate for the patient. For many forms of

Table C-3   Criteria for further evaluation*

- Uncertain diagnosis and inability to develop a reasonable management plan based on the basic diagnostic evaluation. Uncertainty in diagnosis may occur when there is lack of correlation between symptoms and clinical findings.
- Failure to respond to the patient's satisfaction to an adequate therapeutic trial, and the patient is interested in pursuing further therapy.
- Consideration of surgical intervention, particularly if previous surgery failed or the patient is a high surgical risk.
- Hematuria without infection.
- The presence of other comorbid conditions, such as
  Incontinence associated with recurrent symptomatic UTI
  Persistent symptoms of difficult bladder emptying
  History of previous anti-incontinence surgery or radical pelvic surgery
  Beyond hymen and symptomatic pelvic prolapse
  Prostate nodule, asymmetry, or other suspicion of prostate cancer
  Abnormal PVR urine
  Neurologic condition, such as multiple sclerosis and spinal cord lesions or injury.

*Some patients who meet the criteria may not be appropriate for further evaluation and treatment if such evaluation and/or treatment is not desired by or feasible for the patient.

UI, behavioral techniques meet these criteria. Table C-4a, C-4b, and C-4c outline the major treatment options.

Other Measures and Supportive Devices

Other measures and supportive devices in the management of UI include intermittent catheterization, indwelling urethral catheterization, suprapubic catheters, external collection systems, penile compression devices, pelvic organ support devices, and protective pads and garments. Recommendations for the use of these measures and devices are included in Table C-5.

Management of Chronic Intractable UI

Although many persons can benefit from behavioral, pharmacologic, or surgical interventions for UI, many others cannot. Typically, these persons reside in long-term care facilities or are home-bound and have cognitive or physical impairments that prevent them from learning or performing behavioral methods. In addition, these individuals often cannot tolerate or would not benefit from pharmacologic or surgical interventions.

The care of persons with chronic UI should include attention to toileting schedules, fluid and dietary intake, strategies to decrease

Table C-4a   Management options: behavioral interventions

Type of Intervention	Definition	Target Population
Toileting Programs		
Scheduled toileting/ habit training	■ Timed scheduled voiding ■ Habit training scheduled to match patient's voiding habits ■ Caregiver dependent	■ Cognitively impaired ■ Functionally disabled ■ Incomplete bladder emptying ■ Caregiver dependent
Prompted voiding	■ Scheduled voiding that requires prompting from caregiver ■ Caregiver dependent	■ Functionally able to use toilet or toileting device ■ Able to feel urge sensation ■ Able to request toileting assistance ■ Availability of caregiver
Bladder training	■ Systematic ability to delay voiding through the use of urge inhibition ■ Active rehabilitation and education techniques	■ Cognitively intact ■ Ability to discern urge sensation ■ Cognitively able to understand or learn how to inhibit urge ■ Able to toilet themselves or with assistance
Pelvic Muscle Rehabilitation		
Pelvic muscle exercises	■ Planned, active exercises of pelvic muscles to increase periurethral muscle strength ■ Active rehabilitation and education techniques	■ Able to identify and contract pelvic muscles ■ Compliance with instructions
Vaginal weight training	■ Active retention of increasing vaginal weights to induce increased pelvic muscle strength ■ Active rehabilitation and education techniques ■ Contraindication: Pelvic organ prolapse	■ Cognitively intact ■ Compliant with instructions ■ Must be able to stand ■ Must have sufficient pelvic floor strength to be able to contract muscle and retain lightest weight
Biofeedback	■ Method that uses electronic or mechanical instruments to display information about neuromuscular and/or bladder activity, particularly with pelvic muscle exercises. Can be used in association with other programs. ■ Active rehabilitation and education techniques	■ Ability to understand analog or digital signals using auditory or visual display ■ Motivated persons who are able to learn voluntary control through observation of the biofeedback ■ Health care provider who can appropriately assess the UI problem and provide behavioral interventions

Table C-4a   Management options: behavioral interventions—cont'd

Type of Intervention	Definition	Target Population
Electrical stimulation	■ Application of electrical current to sacral and pudendal afferent fibers via intra-anal and/or intravaginal electrodes to inhibit bladder instability and improve striated sphincter and levator ani contractility and efficiency ■ Active rehabilitation and education techniques ■ Contraindication: Vaginal soreness, constipation, hematoma with needle stimulation	■ Useful as adjunct therapy in identification of pelvic muscles ■ Ability to discern stimulation

urine loss at night, use of the most absorbent and skin-friendly protective garments, and prevention and early treatment of skin breakdown.

Continence status can be categorized as follows:

- *Independent continence* describes those who are able to maintain continence without assistance.
- *Dependent continence* applies to persons who are physically or mentally impaired and are kept dry through the efforts of others.
- *Social continence* applies to those incapable of maintaining continence independently or through regular toileting by caregivers and who depend on absorbent products and other measures to contain or collect urine leakage.

Assessment

The basic evaluation checklist should be followed for the assessment of patients with suspected chronic UI.

In addition, the Health Care Financing Administration requires standardized comprehensive assessment and screening of nursing home residents using the instrument known as the Minimum Data Set on admission and quarterly during their stay in a facility. When a patient is incontinent or has an indwelling catheter, a Resident Assessment Profile is also performed to determine the cause, chronicity, and type of UI experienced by the patient. A stress test and evaluation of PVR volume are recommended, and general guide-

Table C-4b   Management options: pharmacologic interventions

Classification	Examples (Usual Oral Dosages)	Action	Indications	Side Effects and Complications
Anticholinergic agents TCAs	Oxybutinin (2.5-5 mg tid or qid), propantheline (7.5-30 mg at least tid), dicyclomine (10-20 mg tid) Imipramine, doxepin, desipramine, nortriptyline (25-100 mg/day)	Reduction or inhibition of involuntary detrusor contraction and increase in bladder capacity.	Urge incontinence	Dry mouth, visual disturbances, constipation, dry skin. Should not be used in cases of obstruction.
Alpha-adrenergic agents	Phenylpropanolamine (25-100 mg bid), pseudoephedrine (15-30 mg tid), ephedrine, epinephrine, norepinephrine	Alpha-adrenergic stimulation increases striated and/or smooth muscle tone increasing urethral resistance.	Stress incontinence	Anxiety, insomnia, agitation, respiratory difficulty, sweating, cardioarrhythmia, hypertension. Should not be used in cases of obstructive syndromes and/or hypertensive disease.
Estrogen replacement agents	Conjugated estrogens (0.3-1.25 mg/day orally or 2 g or fraction/day vaginally)	Stimulation of squamous epithelium; other mechanisms not known.	Stress or mixed incontinence	Should not be used in cases of suspected or confirmed cancer of the breast, undiagnosed vaginal bleeding, suspected or confirmed cancer of the uterus. Progesterone should be given if the patient has not had hysterectomy. Other contraindications may apply; individual assessment is important.

Table C-4c   Management options: surgical management

Type of UI	Cause	Treatment
Stress	Hypermobility	Retropubic suspension. Needle endoscopic suspension
	Intrinsic sphincter deficiency	Sling (mostly women). Artificial sphincter. Urethral bulking
Urge	Refractory detrusor instability	Augmentation cystoplasty
Overflow	Obstruction	Relieve obstruction
	Nonobstructive	Intermittent catheterization Other

lines are provided for referral for additional evaluation. A bladder record should be added to determine the frequency and severity of the UI to provide appropriate treatment. Formal assessment of cognitive function may be helpful in selecting appropriate behavioral intervention, but a short trial is pivotal to assess responsiveness to a particular intervention.

The combination of the Resident Assessment Profile and application of the above definitions can help in evaluating residents and for selecting appropriate intervention. Although such evaluation tools are not mandated for home care agencies, the assessment and management of UI among homebound individuals require a systematic, consistent approach as outlined in the basic evaluation checklist.

Interventions for Chronic UI

Before a patient is classified as suffering from chronic intractable UI, the most appropriate intervention should be attempted. This guideline and most experts suggest that if the patient has stress, urge, or mixed UI, low-risk behavioral treatments should be attempted first if there are no contraindications. Persons with overflow UI who do not have correctable obstruction may be candidates for intermittent catheterization. Some patients may be candidates for surgical or pharmacologic interventions. However, side effects and complications of these treatments are major factors to consider in the treatment of dependent homebound or long-term care patients.

Specific recommendations for the management of chronic UI are provided in Table C-5.

Text continued on p. 386

Table C-5   Summary of guideline recommendations

The ratings in parentheses indicate the scientific evidence supporting each recommendation according to the following scale:

A. The recommendation statement is supported by scientific evidence from properly designed and implemented controlled trials providing statistical results that consistently support the guideline statement.

B. The recommendation statement is supported by scientific evidence from properly designed and implemented clinical series that support the guideline statement.

C. The recommendation statement is supported by expert opinion.

	Recommendation	Recommendation Against
Basic evaluation	History (B). Physical examination (B). Measurement of PVR volume (B). Urinalysis (B). Direct visualization (C).	
Supplementary laboratory tests	Blood testing (BUN, creatinine, glucose, and calcium) if compromised renal function is suspected or if polyuria (in the absence of diuretics) is present (C).	Urine cytology (B).
Risk factors/ prevention	Identify risk factors associated with UI and attempt to modify them (B). Teach women PMEs (C). Teach exercises to strengthen pelvic floor muscles (C).	Specialized tests as part of the basic evaluation (B).
Further evaluation	For patients who fail trial management after the basic evaluation or who are not appropriate for treatment based on presumptive diagnosis (C).	
Urodynamic tests	Simple cystometry for detecting detrusor compliance and contractibility, measuring PVR, and determining capacity (A). More complex cystometric tests appropriate in other situations (B). Urethral sphincteric evaluation (e.g., pressure transmission ratio, leak point pressure) when appropriate (C). Attempt to reproduce the patient's symptoms when performing urodynamic studies (C).	

Table C-5   Summary of guideline recommendations—cont'd

	Recommendation	Recommendation Against
Endoscopic	Cystoscopy when the following are present: sterile hematuria or pyuria (B); when urodynamics fail to duplicate symptoms (C); new onset of irritative voiding symptoms, bladder pain, recurrent cystitis, or suspected foreign body (B).	Cystoscopy in the basic evaluation of UI (B).
Imaging tests	Radiographic ultrasonographic, and other imaging tests should be used for the evaluation of anatomic conditions associated with UI when clinically needed (C).	
Behavioral Interventions		
Routine/scheduled toileting	Routine/scheduled toileting on a consistent schedule for patients who cannot participate in independent toileting (C).	
Habit training	Habit training for patients for whom a natural voiding pattern can be determined (B).	
Prompted voiding	Prompted voiding in patients who can learn to recognize some degree of bladder fullness or the need to void, or who can ask for assistance or respond when prompted to toilet. Patients who are appropriate for prompted voiding may not have sufficient cognitive ability to participate in other, more complex behavioral therapies (A).	
Bladder training	Bladder training strongly recommended for management of urge (DI) and mixed incontinence. Also recommended for management of stress urinary incontinence (SUI) (A).	

Continued

Table C-5   Summary of guideline recommendations—cont'd

	Recommendation	Recommendation Against
Pelvic muscle rehabilitation	PMEs strongly recommended for women with SUI (A). PMEs recommended in men and women in conjunction with bladder training for urge incontinence (B). PMEs may also benefit men who develop UI following prostatectomy (C). Pelvic muscle rehabilitation and bladder inhibition using biofeedback therapy for patients with stress UI, urge UI, and mixed UI (A). Vaginal weight training for SUI in premenopausal women (B). Pelvic floor electrical stimulation has been shown to decrease incontinence in women with SUI (B) and may be useful for urge and mixed incontinence (B).	
Pharmacologic Treatment		
Urge incontinence	The following pharmacologic agents are reported to be useful in urge incontinence as observed in clinical practice (B) ■ Anticholinergic agents—oxybutynin, dicyclomine hydrochloride, and propantheline. ■ TCAs—imipramine, doxepin, desipramine, and nortriptyline. Anticholinergic agents as first-line pharmacologic therapy for patients with DI (A). Oxybutynin is the anticholinergic agent of choice. The recommended dosage is 2.5-5 mg taken orally three or four times per day (A).	Flavoxate for the treatment of patients with DI (A). NSAIDs for the primary treatment of DI (C).

Table C-5   Summary of guideline recommendations—cont'd

	Recommendation	Recommendation Against
	Propantheline is a second-line anticholinergic agent in the treatment of patients with DI who can tolerate the full dose. The recommended doses are 7.5-30 mg administered in the fasting state three to five times per day; higher doses (15-60 mg qid) may be required (B).	
	The use of TCAs should be reserved for carefully evaluated patients. The usual oral dosages are 10-25 mg initially administered one to three times per day, but less frequent administration is usually possible because of the long half-life of these drugs. The daily total dose is usually 25-100 mg (B).	
Stress incontinence	PPA or pseudoephedrine as first-line pharmacologic therapy for women with SUI who have no contraindications for its use, particularly hypertension. The recommended dosage for PPA is 25-100 mg in sustained-release form, administered orally, twice daily (A). The usual dose of pseudoephedrine is 15-30 mg tid.	Propranolol or other beta-blockers for treatment of SUI because of lack of clinical experience and clinical studies (C).
	Estrogen (oral or vaginal) as an adjunctive pharmacologic agent for postmenopausal women with SUI or mixed incontinence. Conjugated estrogen is usually administered either orally (0.3-1.25 mg/day) or vaginally (2 g or fraction/day). Progestin (e.g., medroxyprogesterone 2.5-10 mg/day) may be given continuously or intermittently (B).	
	Combination therapy of oral or vaginal estrogens and PPA in the treatment of SUI in postmenopausal women when initial single-drug therapy has proven inadequate (A).	

Continued

Table C-5   Summary of guideline recommendations—cont'd

	Recommendation	Recommendation Against
	Imipramine as an alternative pharmacologic therapy for SUI when first-line agents have proven unsatisfactory (C).	
Surgical Treatment		
Stress incontinence	Surgery is recommended for treatment of stress incontinence in men and women and may be recommended as first-line treatment for appropriately selected patients and those who are unable to comply with other nonsurgical therapies (B).	
Hypermobility in women	Retropubic or needle suspension for women with hypermobility when SUI is the primary indication for surgery. On the basis of greater efficacy, these procedures are recommended over anterior vaginal repair for hypermobility (B).	
Intrinsic sphincter deficiency (ISD) in women	Sling procedures for women who have ISD with coexisting hypermobility or as first-line treatment for ISD (B). Periurethral bulking injections as first-line treatment for women with ISD who do not have coexisting hypermobility (B). Artificial sphincter for ISD patients who are unable to perform intermittent catheterization and have severe SUI that is unresponsive to other surgical treatments. Because of the high complication rate, this treatment is rarely used as primary therapy (B).	
ISD in men	Periurethral bulking injections as a first-line surgical treatment for men with ISD (B). Artificial sphincter for ISD during the 6 months after prostatectomy. Behavioral intervention should also be tried during this period (B).	

Table C-5   Summary of guideline recommendations—cont'd

	Recommendation	Recommendation Against
Urge incontinence: detrusor instability	Augmentation intestinocystoplasty for those with intractable, severe bladder instability or for those with bladders that have poor compliance when the patient is unresponsive to other nonsurgical therapies (B). Urinary diversion is recommended in severe intractable cases of detrusor instability that is unresponsive to other therapies (C).	
Overflow incontinence: bladder neck or urethral obstruction	Symptoms of overflow or incontinence secondary to obstruction should be addressed with a surgical procedure to relieve the obstruction (B). Intermittent catheterization or an indwelling catheter in patients who are not candidates for surgery (C).	The panel found no evidence to support the use of urethral dilation for treating incontinence in women, although it may be useful in the extremely rare cases of primary obstruction (C). Internal urethrotomy for treating urethral obstruction in women (C).

Other Measures and Supportive Devices

	Recommendation	Recommendation Against
Intermittent catheterization	Intermittent catheterization (IC) as a supportive measure for patients with spinal cord injury, persistent UI, or with chronic urinary retention secondary to underactive or partially obstructed bladder (B). Clean technique for IC in young, male, neurologically impaired individuals (B). Sterile technique for IC for elderly patients and patients with compromised immune system (C).	Routine use of long-term suppressive therapy with antibiotics in patients with chronic, clean IC (B). In high-risk populations, for example, those with internal prosthesis or those who are immuno-suppressed due to age or disease, the use of antibiotic therapy for asymptomatic bacteriuria must be individually reviewed (C).
Indwelling catheters	As a supportive measure for patients whose incontinence is caused by obstruction and for whom other interventions are not feasible (B). Incontinent patients who are terminally ill or for patients with pressure ulcers as short-term treatment (B).	

Continued

Table C-5   Summary of guideline recommendations—cont'd

	Recommendation	Recommendation Against
	In severely impaired individuals in whom alternative interventions are not an option and when a patient lives alone and a caregiver is unavailable to provide other supportive measures (C).	
Suprapubic catheters	For short-term use following gynecologic, urologic, and other surgery, or as an alternative to long-term catheter use (B).	In persons with chronic unstable bladder (DI, DH) and ISD (B).
External collection systems	For incontinent men and women ■ who have adequate bladder emptying. ■ who have intact genital skin. ■ in whom other therapies have failed or are not appropriate (C).	
Penile compression devices	Penile compression devices are known to be used in clinical practice in the treatment of UI. No scientific literature was found to support the use of these devices. The panel recognizes the temporary use of penile compression devices in males in selected circumstances under the supervision of a health care provider (C).	
Pelvic organ support devices	Pessaries for women who have symptomatic pelvic organ prolapse (C).	Data are not available to recommend or discourage the use of pessaries for the treatment of UI in women (C).
Absorbent products	During evaluation (C). As an adjunct to other therapy (C). For long-term care of patients with chronic, intractable UI (C).	
Long-Term Management of Chronic Intractable UI		
Physical and environmental alterations	Caregiver assessment of the environment in which the elderly or disabled patient resides. Simple alterations or the addition of toileting or ambulation devices to eliminate or reduce episodes of involuntary urine loss (C).	

Table C-5   Summary of guideline recommendations—cont'd

	Recommendation	Recommendation Against
Fluid and dietary management	Strategies that maintain or improve mobility to prevent or reduce incontinent episodes in the frail elderly (B). A bowel regimen based on adequate fiber and fluid intake. Elimination of bowel impaction and consequent pressure on the bladder and urethra as necessary first steps in the treatment of chronic UI (C).	
Management of nocturia	Preventive measures to decrease night-time voids. Simple electronic urine detection devices for more efficient and effective patient monitoring of night-time urine loss (B).	
Interventions for protection and comfort	Most absorbent and skin-friendly products. However, no scientific literature was found to guide in selection of the most effective product (C). Intermittent catheterization preferable to indwelling catheters for the management of urinary retention and overflow incontinence (B). Suprapubic catheters as alternative for indwelling urethral catheters when patient choice or circumstances require the use of a bladder drainage device (B).	
Skin care	Standard measures of cleansing the skin immediately before and after urine loss (B). Most absorbent and skin-friendly pads and garments for protection from skin damage (C).	

Continued

Table C-5   Summary of guideline recommendations—cont'd

	Recommendation	Recommendation Against
Public and Professional Education		
	Comprehensive and multi-disciplinary patient education about incontinence and all management alternatives (C).	
	More research to test the effectiveness of patient education activities (C).	
	Inclusion of education about UI evaluation and treatment in the basic curricula of undergraduate and graduate training programs of all health care providers (C).	
	Continuing education programs on UI for health care providers (C).	

Public and Professional Education

Because of the social stigma of UI, many sufferers do not even report the problem to a health care provider. In addition, when it is reported, many physicians and nurses, who need to be educated in this area, fail to pursue investigation of UI. As a result, this medical problem is vastly underdiagnosed and underreported.

One of the major areas for which the guideline provides practice recommendations is education, both of the public and of health care providers. The guideline calls for continued efforts to educate health care providers about this condition so that they are sufficiently knowledgeable to diagnose and treat it. It recommends that the public be advised to report incontinence problems once they occur and be informed that incontinence is not inevitable or shameful but is a treatable or at least manageable condition.

UI outcome measures need to be developed so that nursing home surveyors are better able to assess the effectiveness of interventions for UI in this setting.

Selected Bibliography

Appell RA: Collagen injection therapy for urinary incontinence, *Urol Clin North Am* 21(1):177, 1994.

Awad SA, Gajewski JB, Katz NO et al: Final diagnosis and therapeutic implications of mixed symptoms of urinary incontinence in women, *Urology* 34:352, 1992.

Baker KR, Drutz HP: Age as a risk factor in major genitourinary surgery, *Can J Surg* 35:188, 1992.

Beck RP, McCormick S, Nordstrom L: A 25 year experience with 519 anterior colporrhaphy procedures, *Obstet Gynecol* 78:1011, 1991.

Benderev TV: Anchor fixation and other modifications of endoscopic bladder neck suspensions, *Urology* 40:409, 1992.

Bump RC, McClish DM: Cigarette smoking and pure genuine stress incontinence of urine. A comparison of risk factors and determinants between smokers and nonsmokers, *Am J Obstet Gynecol* 170(2):579, 1994.

Burgio KL, Matthews KA, Engel BT: Prevalence, incidence and correlates of urinary incontinence in healthy, middle-aged women, *J Urol* 146:1255, 1991.

Burgio KL, Stutzman RE, Engel BT: Behavioral training for post-prostatectomy urinary incontinence, *J Urol* 141:303, 1989.

Burgio LD, McCormick KA, Scheve AS, et al: The effects of changing prompted voiding schedules in the treatment of incontinence in nursing home residents, *J Am Geriatr Soc* 42(3):315, 1994.

Burns PA, Pranifoff K, Nochajski TH et al: A comparison of effectiveness of biofeedback and pelvic muscle exercise treatment of stress-incontinence in older community-dwelling women, *J Gerontol* 48(4):167, 1993.

Castleden CM, Duffin HM, Gulati RS: Double-blind study of imipramine and placebo for incontinence due to bladder instability, *Age Ageing* 15(5):299, 1986.

Colling J, Ouslander J, Hadley BJ et al: The effects of patterned urge response toileting (PURT) on urinary incontinence among nursing home residents, *J Am Geriatr Soc* 40:135, 1992.

Diokno AC: Diagnostic categories of incontinence and the role of urodynamic testing, *J Am Geriatr Soc* 38(3):300, 1990.

Fantl JA, Cardozo L, McClish DK: Hormones and Urogenital Therapy Committee. Estrogen therapy in the management of urinary incontinence in postmenopausal women: a meta-analysis: first report of the hormones and urogenital therapy committee, *Obstet Gynecol* 83:12, 1994.

Fantl JA, Wyman JF, McClish DK et al: Efficacy of bladder training in older women with urinary incontinence, *JAMA* 265(5):609, 1991.

Ferguson K, McKey PL, Bishop KR et al: Stress urinary incontinence: effect of pelvic muscle exercise, *Obstet Gynecol* 73:671, 1990.

Foldspang A, Mommsen S, Lam FW et al: Parity as a correlate of adult female urinary incontinence prevalence, *J Epidemiol Community Health* 46:595, 1992.

Fonda A: *Improving management of urinary incontinence in geriatric centers and nursing homes.* Victorian Geriatrician Peer Review Group, Australian Clinical Review (Sydney) 10(2):66, 1990.

Godec CJ: Timed voiding: a useful tool in the treatment of urinary incontinence, *Urology* 23(1):97, 1994.

Herzog AR, Fultz NH, Normolle DP et al: Methods used to manage urinary incontinence by older adults in the community, *J Am Geriatr Soc* 37(4):339, 1989.

Hilton P, Tweddell AL, Mayne C: Oral and intravaginal estrogens alone and in combination with alpha-adrenergic stimulation in genuine stress incontinence, *Int Urogynecol J* 1(2):80, 1990.

Hu T, Gabelko K, Weis KA et al: Clinical guidelines and cost implications—the case of urinary incontinence, *Geriatr Nephrol Urol* 4:85, 1994.

Jirovec MM: The impact of daily exercise on the mobility balance and urine control of cognitively impaired nursing home residents, *Int J Nurs Stud* 28(2):145, 1991.

McDowell BJ, Burgio KL, Dombrowski M et al: An interdisciplinary approach to the assessment and behavioral treatment of urinary incontinence in geriatric outpatients, *J Am Geriatr Soc* 40:370, 1992.

McFall SL, Yerkes AM, Belzer JA et al: Urinary incontinence and quality of life in older women: a community demonstration in Oklahoma, *Fam Community Health* 17(1):64, 1994.

McGuire EJ: Disorders of the control of bladder contractility. In Kursh ED, McGuire EJ, eds, *Female urology.* Philadelphia, 1994, Lippincott.

McGuire EJ, Appell RA: Transurethral collagen injection for urinary incontinence, *Urology* 43(4):413, 1994.

Morris JN, Hawes C, Murphy K et al: *Long term care resident assessment instrument training manual,* Baltimore, MD: Health Care Financing Administration, p. 279, 1990.

Nygaard IE, Thompson FL, Svengalis SL et al: Urinary incontinence in elite nulliparous athletes, *Obstet Gynecol* 84(2):182, 1994.

Olah KS, Bridges N, Denning J et al: The conservative management of patients with symptoms of stress incontinence: a randomized, prospective study comparing weighted vaginal cones and interferential therapy, *Am J Obstet Gynecol* 162(1):87, 1990.

Ouslander JG, Greengold B, Chen S: External catheter use and urinary tract infections among incontinent male nursing home patients, *J Am Geriatr Soc* 35:1063, 1987.

Palmer MH, German PS, Ouslander JG: Risk factors for urinary incontinence one year after nursing home admission, *Res Nurs Health* 14:405, 1991.

Resnick NM, Baumann MM: A national assessment strategy for urinary incontinence in nursing homes, *Neurourol Urodyn* 9:411, 1990.

Sand PK, Brubaker LT, Novak T: Standing incremental cystometry as a screening method for detrusor instability, *Obstet Gynecol* 77:453, 1991.

Sand PK, Richardson DA, Staskin DR et al: Pelvic floor electrical stimulation in the treatment of genuine stress incontinence: a multicenter, placebo-controlled trial, *Am J Obstet Gynecol* 173:72, 1995.

Schnelle JF, Newman DR, White M et al: Maintaining continence in NH residents through the application of industrial quality control, *Gerontologist* 33:114, 1993.

Shumaker SA, Wyman JF, Uebersax JS et al: Health-related quality-of-life measures for women with urinary incontinence—the incontinence impact questionnaire and the urogenital distress inventory, *Qual Life Res* 3(5):291, 1994.

Sowell VA, Schnelle JF, Hu TW et al: A cost comparison of five methods of managing urinary incontinence, *Q Rev Biol* Dec; 411, 1987.

Strahan GW: *An overview of home health and hospice care patients: preliminary data from the 1993 National Home and Hospice Care Survey.* Advance data from Vital and Health Statistics; No. 256. Hyattsville (MD): National Center for Health Statistics, 1994.

Thuroff JW, Bunke B, Ebner A et al: Randomized, double-blind, multicenter trial on treatment of frequency, urgency and incontinence related to detrusor hyperactivity: oxybutynin versus propantheline versus placebo, *J Urol* 145(4):813, 1991.

Topper JR, Holliday PJ, Fernie GR: Bladder volume estimation in the elderly using a portable ultrasound-based measurement device, *J Med Eng Technol* 17(3):99, 1993.

Walter S, Kjaergaard B, Lose G et al: Stress urinary incontinence in postmenopausal women treated with oral estrogen (estriol) and an alpha-adrenoceptor-stimulating agent (phenylpropanolamine): a randomized double-blind placebo-controlled study, *Int Urogynecol J* 1(2):74, 1990.

Warren JW, Muncie HL, Hall-Craggs M: Acute pyelonephritis associated with bacteriuria during long-term catheterization: a prospective clinico-pathological study, *J Infect Dis* 158(6):1341, 1988.

Wells T, Brink C, Diokno A et al: Pelvic muscle exercise for stress urinary incontinence in elderly women, *J Am Geriatr Soc* 39:785, 1991.

Wyman JF, Choi SC, Harkins SW et al: The urinary diary in evaluation of urinary incontinence in women: a test retest analysis, *Obstet Gynecol* 71(6 pt. 1):812, 1988.

Appendix D
Pressure Ulcers
in Adults: Prediction
and Prevention

Pressure ulcers are serious problems that can lead to pain, a longer hospital stay, and a slower recovery. Fortunately, most can be prevented, and stage I pressure ulcers (nonblanchable erythema of intact skin) that do form need not worsen in most circumstances. However, even the most vigilant nursing care may not prevent the development and worsening of pressure ulcers in some very high-risk individuals. In those cases, intensive therapy must be aimed at reducing risk factors, preventive measures, and treatment.

The purpose of this appendix is to help clinicians identify adults at risk of developing pressure ulcers and to define early interventions for prevention; these guidelines may also be used to treat stage I pressure ulcers. However, these guidelines do not apply to infants and children, to clients with existing stage II or greater pressure ulcers, or to individuals who are fully mobile.

Recommendations target four goals: (1) to identify individuals at risk who need preventive care and the specific factors placing them at risk; (2) to maintain and improve tissue tolerance to pressure in order to prevent injury; (3) to protect against the adverse effects of external mechanical forces (pressure, friction, and

From Panel on the Prediction and Prevention of Pressure Ulcers in Adults. Pressure ulcers in adults: prediction and prevention. In *Quick reference guide for clinicians,* AHCPR Publication No. 92-0050, Rockville, Md, 1992, Agency for Health Care Policy and Research, Public Health Service, US Department of Health and Human Services.

shear); and (4) to reduce the incidence of pressure ulcers by providing educational programs.

A pressure ulcer is defined as any lesion caused by unrelieved pressure that results in damage to underlying tissue. Pressure ulcers usually occur over bony prominences, and they are graded or staged to classify the degree of tissue damage observed. The staging of pressure ulcers recommended for use by AHCPR is consistent with the recommendations of the National Pressure Ulcer Advisory Panel (NPUAP):

- **Stage I.** Nonblanchable erythema of intact skin; the heralding lesion of skin ulceration. NOTE: Reactive hyperemia can normally be expected to be present for one-half to three-fourths as long as the pressure occluded blood flow to the area; it should not be confused with a stage I pressure ulcer.
- **Stage II.** Partial-thickness skin loss involving epidermis and/or dermis. The ulcer is superficial and presents clinically as an abrasion, blister, or shallow crater.
- **Stage III.** Full-thickness skin loss involving damage or necrosis of subcutaneous tissue that may extend down to, but not through, underlying fascia. The ulcer presents clinically as a deep crater with or without undermining of adjacent tissue.
- **Stage IV.** Full-thickness skin loss with extensive destruction, tissue necrosis, or damage to muscle, bone, or supporting structures (for example, tendon or joint capsule). NOTE: Undermining and sinus tracts may also be associated with stage IV pressure ulcers.

Staging definitions recognize these limitations:

- Assessment of stage I pressure ulcers may be difficult in patients with darkly pigmented skin.
- When eschar is present, accurate staging of the pressure ulcer is not possible until the eschar has sloughed or the wound has been debrided.

These guidelines are intended for clinicians who examine and treat persons at risk of developing pressure ulcers. These clinicians include family physicians, internists, geriatricians, dietitians, occupational and physical therapists, nurses, and nurse practitioners working in a variety of health care settings, such as acute care, rehabilitation, geriatric care, and home- and community-based settings.

After an extensive review of the scientific literature, the panel used the following criteria to grade the evidence supporting each recommendation:

A. There is good research-based evidence to support the recommendation.
B. There is fair research-based evidence to support the recommendation.
C. The recommendation is based on expert opinion and panel consensus.

Risk Assessment Tools and Risk Factors

Goal: To identify individuals at risk who need preventive care and the specific factors placing them at risk.

Bed- and chair-bound individuals or those with impaired ability to reposition should be assessed for additional factors that increase risk for developing pressure ulcers. These factors include immobility, incontinence, nutritional factors (e.g., inadequate dietary intake and impaired nutritional status), and altered level of consciousness. Individuals should be assessed on admission to acute care and rehabilitation hospitals, nursing homes, home care programs, and other health care facilities. A systematic risk assessment can be accomplished by using a validated risk assessment tool such as the Braden Scale or Norton Scale. (Table 1 contains the Norton Scale. See Fig. 5-3 in Chapter 5 for the Braden Scale.) Pressure ulcer risk should be reassessed periodically. *(Strength of evidence = A)* All assessments of risk should be documented. *(Strength of evidence = C)*

Skin Care and Early Treatment

Goal: To maintain and improve tissue tolerance to pressure in order to prevent injury.

1. At least once a day, all individuals at risk should have a systematic skin inspection during which particular attention is paid to the bony prominences. Results of skin inspection should be documented. *(Strength of evidence = C)*
2. Skin should be cleansed immediately after soiling and at routine intervals. The frequency of skin cleansing should be individualized according to need and/or client preference. Avoid hot water, and use a mild cleansing agent that minimizes irritation and dryness of the skin. During the cleans-

Table 1   Norton Scale

Name	Date	Physical Condition		Mental Condition		Activity		Mobility		Incontinent		Total Score
		Good	4	Alert	4	Ambulant	4	Full	4	Not	4	
		Fair	3	Apathetic	3	Walk/help	3	Slightly limited	3	Occasional	3	
		Poor	2	Confused	2	Chairbound	2	Very limited	2	Usually/urine	2	
		Very bad	1	Stupor	1	Stupor	1	Immobile	1	Doubly	1	

From Norton D, McLaren R, Exton-Smith AN: *An investigation of geriatric nursing problems in the hospital,* London, 1962, National Corporation for the Care of Old People (now the Centre for Policy on Ageing). Reprinted with permission.

ing process, care should be used to minimize the force and friction applied to the skin. *(Strength of evidence = C)*

3. Minimize environmental factors leading to skin drying, such as low humidity (less than 40%) and exposure to cold. Dry skin should be treated with moisturizers. *(Strength of evidence = C)*

4. Avoid massage over bony prominences. Current evidence suggests that massage over bony prominences may be harmful. *(Strength of evidence = B)*

5. Minimize skin exposure to moisture caused by incontinence, perspiration, or wound drainage. When these sources of moisture cannot be controlled, use underpads or briefs that are made of materials that absorb moisture and present a quick-drying surface to the skin. Topical agents that act as barriers to moisture can also be used. *(Strength of evidence = C)*

6. Skin injury caused by friction and shear forces should be minimized through proper positioning, transferring, and turning techniques. In addition, friction injuries may be reduced by the use of lubricants (such as corn starch and creams), protective films (such as transparent film dressings and skin sealants), protective dressings (such as hydrocolloids), and protective padding. *(Strength of evidence = C)*

7. When apparently well-nourished individuals develop an inadequate dietary intake of protein or calories, caregivers should first attempt to discover the factors compromising intake and offer support with eating. Other nutritional supplements or support may be needed. If dietary intake remains inadequate and if consistent with overall goals of therapy, more aggressive nutritional intervention such as enteral or parenteral feedings should be considered. *(Strength of evidence = C)*

   For nutritionally compromised individuals, a plan of nutritional support and/or supplementation should be implemented that meets individual needs and is consistent with the overall goals of therapy. *(Strength of evidence = C)*

8. If the potential exists for improving the individual's mobility and activity status, rehabilitation efforts should be instituted if consistent with the overall goals of therapy. Maintaining current activity level, mobility, and range of motion is an appropriate goal for most individuals. *(Strength of evidence = C)*

9. Interventions and outcomes should be monitored and documented. *(Strength of evidence = C)*

Mechanical Loading and Support Surfaces

Goal: To protect against the adverse effects of external mechanical forces (pressure, friction, and shear).

1. Any bedridden individual at risk for developing pressure ulcers should be repositioned at least every 2 hours if consistent with overall client goals. A written schedule for systematically turning and repositioning the individual should be used. *(Strength of evidence = B)*

2. For individuals in bed, positioning devices such as pillows or foam wedges should be used to keep bony prominences (such as knees or ankles) from direct contact with one another, according to a written plan. *(Strength of evidence = C)*

3. Individuals in bed who are completely immobile should have a care plan that includes the use of devices that totally relieve pressure on the heels, most commonly by raising the heels off the bed. Do not use donut-type devices. *(Strength of evidence = C)*

4. When the side-lying position is used in bed, avoid positioning directly on the trochanter. *(Strength of evidence = C)*

5. Maintain the head of the bed at the lowest degree of elevation consistent with medical conditions and other restrictions. Limit the amount of time the head of the bed is elevated. *(Strength of evidence = C)*

6. Use lifting devices such as a trapeze or bed linen to move (rather than drag) individuals in bed who cannot assist during transfers and position changes. *(Strength of evidence = C)*

7. When lying in bed, any individual at risk for developing pressure ulcers should be placed on a pressure-reducing device, such as foam, static air, alternating air, gel, or water mattresses. *(Strength of evidence = B)*

8. Any person at risk for developing a pressure ulcer should avoid uninterrupted sitting in any chair or wheelchair. The individual should be repositioned, shifting the points under pressure at least every hour, or be put back to bed, depending on overall client management goals. Individuals who

are able should be taught to shift weight every 15 minutes. *(Strength of evidence = C)*

9. For chair-bound individuals, the use of a pressure-reducing device (such as those made of foam, gel, air, or a combination) is indicated. Do not use donut-type devices. *(Strength of evidence = C)*

10. When positioning chair-bound individuals, postural alignment, distribution of weight, balance and stability, and pressure relief should be considered. *(Strength of evidence = C)*

11. A written plan for the use of positioning devices and schedules may be helpful for chair-bound individuals. *(Strength of evidence = C)*

Education

Goal: To reduce the incidence of pressure ulcers by providing educational programs.

1. Educational programs for the prevention of pressure ulcers should be structured, organized, and comprehensive, and directed at all levels of health care providers, clients, and families or caregivers. *(Strength of evidence = A)*

2. The educational program for prevention of pressure ulcers should include information on the following items: *(Strength of evidence = B)*
   - The etiology of and risk factors for pressure ulcers
   - Risk assessment tools and their application
   - Skin assessment
   - Selection and/or use of support surfaces
   - Development and implementation of an individualized program of skin care
   - Demonstration of positioning to decrease risk of tissue breakdown
   - Instruction on accurate documentation of pertinent data

3. The educational program should identify those persons responsible for pressure ulcer prevention, describe each person's role, and be appropriate to the audience in terms of level of information presented and expected participation. The educational program should be updated on a regular basis to incorporate new and existing techniques or technologies. *(Strength of evidence = C)*

4. Educational programs should be developed, implemented, and evaluated using principles of adult learning. Programs must have built-in mechanisms such as quality assurance standards and audits to evaluate their effectiveness in preventing pressure ulcers. *(Strength of evidence = C)*

Algorithm

The algorithm that follows was developed as a visual display of the conceptual organization, procedural flow, decision points, and preferred management path previously discussed. It begins at the point of admission to an acute care hospital, rehabilitation hospital, nursing home, home care program, or other health care facility or program. Numbers in the algorithm refer to the annotations that follow.

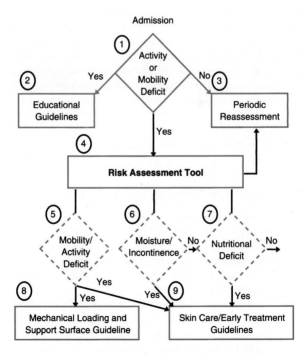

Pressure Ulcer Prediction and Prevention Algorithm

1. **Activity or mobility deficit.** Bed- or chair-bound individuals or those whose ability to reposition is impaired should be considered at risk for pressure ulcers. Identification of additional risk factors (immobility, moisture/incontinence, and nutritional deficit) should be undertaken to direct specific preventive treatment regimes.

2. **Educational program.** Educational programs for the prevention of pressure ulcers should be structured, organized, and comprehensive and directed at all levels of health care providers, clients, and family or caregivers.

3. **Reassessment.** Active, mobile individuals should be periodically reassessed for changes in activity and mobility status. The frequency of reassessment depends on client status and institutional policy.

4. **Risk assessment tools.** Clinicians are encouraged to select and use a method of risk assessment that ensures systematic evaluation of individual risk factors. Many risk assessment tools exist, but only the Norton Scale and Braden Scale have been tested extensively. Risk assessment tools include the following risk factors: mobility/activity impairment, moisture/incontinence, and impaired nutrition. Altered level of consciousness (or altered sensory perception) is also identified as a risk factor in most assessment tools. Identification of individual risk factors (Boxes 5 to 7) is helpful in directing care.

5. **Mobility/activity deficit.** (If there is a deficit, see Boxes 8 and 9.)

Mechanical Loading and Support Surfaces

For bed-bound individuals:

- Reposition at least every 2 hours.
- Use pillows or foam wedges to keep bony prominences from direct contact.
- Use devices that totally relieve pressure on the heels. Avoid positioning directly on the trochanter.
- Elevate the head of the bed as little and for as short a time as possible.
- Use lifting devices to move rather than drag individuals during transfers and position changes.
- Place at-risk individuals on a pressure-reducing mattress. *Do not use donut-type devices.*

For chair-bound individuals:
- Reposition at least every hour.
- Have patient shift weight every 15 minutes if able.
- Use pressure-reducing devices for seating surfaces. *Do not use donut-type devices.*
- Consider postural alignment, distribution of weight, balance and stability, and pressure relief when positioning individuals in chairs or wheelchairs.
- Use a written plan.

Skin Care and Early Treatment

- Inspect skin at least once a day.
- Individualize bathing schedule. Avoid hot water. Use a mild cleansing agent.
- Minimize environmental factors such as low humidity and cold air. Use moisturizers for dry skin.
- Avoid massage over bony prominences.
- Use proper positioning, transferring, and turning techniques.
- Use lubricants to reduce friction injuries.
- Institute a rehabilitation program.
- Monitor and document interventions and outcomes.
- 6. **Moisture/incontinence.** If there is moisture or incontinence, see Skin Care and Early Treatment, Guidelines 2, 5 (pp. 385 and 387).
- Cleanse skin at time of soiling.
- Minimize skin exposure to moisture. Assess and treat urinary incontinence. When moisture cannot be controlled, use underpads or briefs that are absorbent and present a quick-drying surface to the skin.
- 7. **Nutritional deficit:** If there is a nutritional deficit, see Skin Care and Early Treatment, Guideline 7 (p. 387).
- Investigate factors that compromise an apparently well-nourished individual's dietary intake (especially protein or calories) and offer him or her support with eating.
- Plan and implement a nutritional support and/or supplementation program for nutritionally compromised individuals.

Risk should be periodically reassessed. Care should be modified according to the level of risk. Frequency of reassessment depends on client status and institutional policy.

Index

A

Abdomen, 244-265
  auscultation, 254
  constipation, 254-265
  esophageal reflux,
    263-264
  four quadrants, 244, 246,
    248-249
  inspection, 253-254
  muscles, 251
  nine anatomic regions, 247
  organs of digestive
    system, 245
  palpation, 258-263
  percussion, 255-258
  signs of nutrient
    deficiency, 72
Abdominal aorta, 251
Abdominal muscles, 251
Abducens nerve, 137, 332
Abduction, 310
Accommodation, 143
Achalasia, 252
Achilles reflex, 347
Acini, 250-251
Acoustic nerve, 333
Acrochordons, 103
Actinic keratosis, 112
Activities of daily
    living, 37-40
Activity, pressure sore
    risk, 106, 387, 391
Acute confusional states, 7-12
  transient urinary
    incontinence, 363
Adduction, 310
Adventitious breath
    sounds, 206-207

Affect, 93
Affective status
    assessment, 41-50
  Beck Depression
    Inventory, 49-51
  Mini-Mental State
    Exam, 44-46
  Short Blessed Test, 47
  Short Portable Mental
    Status Questionnaire,
    42-44
Afterload, 218
Agency for Health Care
    Policy and Research
    staging of pressure
    ulcers, 384
Aging, interrelationship
    between physical and
    psychosocial aspects,
    2-4
Albumin, 358
Alcohol, effects that may
    affect assessment, 36
Alkaline phosphatase, 359
Alpha-adrenergic agents, 365,
    367
Alternating pulse, 228
Alzheimer's disease, 348
Amphiarthrosis, 307
Ampulla, 267
Anal canal, 270
Anal sphincter tone, 302
Anemia
  nutrient deficiency, 74
  oral manifestations, 158
Angiotensin-converting
    enzyme inhibitors, 36
Angle of Louis, 195

Ankle
 range of motion, 321
 reflex, 347
Annulus, 152
Anorexia, 74
Antacids, 36
Anteflexed uterus, 300
Anterior chamber, 134, 142
Anteverted uterus, 297
Anthropometric assessment,
  67-68, 75-87
 height, 76-77
 knee height, 80
 midarm circumference, 80
 mid-upper arm
  circumference, 81
 triceps skinfold
  thickness, 82-85
 weight, 78-79
Antibiotic therapy, oral
  manifestations, 158
Anticholinergic agents
 effects that may affect
  assessment, 36
 urinary incontinence, 365,
  367
Antidepressants, 365
Antihelix, 151
Antihistamines
 effects that may affect
  assessment, 36
 transient urinary
  incontinence, 365
Antiparkinsonian agents
 effects that may affect
  assessment, 36
 transient urinary
  incontinence, 365
Antipsychotic agents
 effects that may affect
  assessment, 36
 transient urinary
  incontinence, 365
Antispasmodics, 365
Antitragus, 151

Anus
 female, 282
 male, 270-271, 274
Anxiety, 17, 21
Anxiolytics, 36
Aorta, 215, 217
Aortic valve, 216
Apathy, 74
Apocrine glands, 109
Appendix, 249
Areola, 180, 181, 183
Arrhythmia, 72
Arterial blood gases, 359
Arterial insufficiency, 230, 231
Arterial pulse
  abnormalities, 228
Arterial system, 223-226
Articular cartilage
  calcification, 305
Articulation
 classification, 307
 general survey, 91
 movement, 310
 range of motion assessment,
  317-322
Ascending colon, 250
Atrial depolarization, 223
Atrioventricular valve, 215,
  216
Atrium, 214
Atrophic urethritis, 363
Atrophic vaginitis, 303, 363
Atrophy, vulvar, 282
Attention, general survey, 92
Attitude of interviewer, 15
Auditory function, 161
Auditory loss, 3
Auricle, 150
Auscultation, 59-61
 abdomen, 254
 chest, 205, 208-209
 heart, 236-240
Axilla, 179, 180
Axillary lines, 196
Axillary tail, 179, 180

B

Babinski reflex, 347
Bacterial plaque, 156-158
Bacterial pneumonia, 8
Balance, 339-341
Ball and socket joint, 307
Ballottement, 58, 324
Bartholin's glands, 278, 285
Basal cell carcinoma, 112
Bathing, 38, 40
Beck Depression Inventory,
    48, 49-51
Bed-bound client
    mechanical loading and
        support surfaces, 391
    position during health
        history interview, 20
    urinary incontinence,
        378-382
Behavioral therapy for urinary
    incontinence, 366
Benign prostatic hyperplasia,
    269-270, 276
Benztropine mesylate, 365
Beta-blockers, 36
Biceps reflex, 346
Bigeminal pulse, 228
Bile, 250
Bimanual examination,
    294-301
Biochemical measurement, 68
Bisferious pulse, 228
Bitot's spot, 71
Bladder, 251
    decompression, 371
Blessed Dementia
        Scale, 41-44, 47
Blood gases, 359
Blood pressure
    classification, 225
    measurement, 227-230
Blood urea nitrogen, 358
Body development, 90
Body fat, 108
Body lice, 114

Body odor, 56-57
Bone
    anatomy and
        physiology, 306
    signs of nutrient
        deficiency, 72
Bony labyrinth, 153
Bounding pulse, 228
Bowel sounds, 254
Brachial plexus, 334
Brachial pulse, 227
Brachioradialis reflex, 346
Braden Scale, 106-107
Bradycardia, 72, 228
Brain, 327-329
Brainstem, 328, 329, 330-331
Breast, 179-193
    inspection, 182-186
    lymphatics, 181-182
    mammary glands, 179-181
    mass, 188, 192
    palpation, 186-191
    review of systems, 31
    self breast exam, 192-193
Breath sounds, 206-207, 209
Bronchial sounds, 209
Bronchophony, 210
Bronchovesicular sounds, 209
Bronchus, 198
Bruising, 70
Bruit, 254, 255
Bulge sign, 324-325
Bulla, 98

C

Calcification of articular
    cartilage, 305
Calcitonin, 122
Calcium channel blockers
    effects that may affect
        assessment, 36
    transient urinary
        incontinence, 365
Calcium laboratory
    values, 359

Candida albicans, 113
  oral infection, 158
  vaginal smear, 293
Carbon dioxide partial
    pressure, 359
Cardiac cycle, 218-219
Cardinal fields of gaze, 139
Cardiovascular disease
  client teaching, 242
  risk factors, 10
Cardiovascular system, 214-243
  anatomy and physiology,
      214-218
  auscultation, 236-240
  blood pressure, 227-230
  cardiac cycle, 218-219
  heart conduction system,
      219-223
  heart sounds, 219, 220-222
  hypertension, 241
  review of systems, 31-32
  risk factors for cardiac
      disease, 242
  signs of nutrient
      deficiency, 72
Caries, 158
Carotid artery, 224, 226
Carotid pulse, 227, 234
Cataract, 145
Cecum, 249-250
Central chemoreceptor, 199
Central nervous system,
    326-348
  Alzheimer's disease, 348
  anatomy and physiology,
      327-338
    brain, 327-329
    brainstem, 330-331
    cranial nerves, 332-333
    sensory dermatomes,
        335-336
    spinal cord, 328, 337-338
  assessment, 338-347
    balance, 339-341
    cranial nerves, 338-339

Central nervous system—cont'd
  assessment—cont'd
    percussion hammer,
        344-345
    reflexes, 343, 345-347
    sensory examination,
        341-343
  review of systems, 34
  signs of nutrient
      deficiency, 73-74
Cerebellum, 328
Cerebral disease, 10
Cerebral function
    assessment, 88-94
Cerebral hemisphere, 327-328
Cerebrum, 327-328
Cerumen, 152
Cervical plexus, 334
Cervical spine range of
    motion, 318
Cervix, 278
  bimanual examination, 295
  speculum examination,
      287-290
Chair-bound patient
  mechanical loading and
      support surfaces,
      391-392
  position during health
      history interview, 18
Cheilosis, 71
Chemoreceptor, 199
Cherry angioma, 103
Chief complaint, 24
Chlamydial enzyme
    immunoassay
    specimen, 293
Chordae tendineae, 216-217
Chronic disease, 4
Cimetidine, 36
Circulation, peripheral,
    223-226
Circumduction, 310
Cirrhosis, 158

Client teaching
  cardiac disease, 242
  constipation, 264-265
  dry skin, 112
  eye care, 148
  fall prevention, 323-324
  hearing loss, 176
  influenza prevention, 212
  oral health care, 177-178
  self breast exam, 192-193
Clinical examination, 69,
    70-74
Clitoris, 278, 283
Cochlea, 153
Cognitive impairment, 7, 12
Cognitive status assessment,
    41-50
  Beck Depression
    Inventory, 49-51
  Mini-Mental State
    Exam, 44-46
  Short Blessed Test, 47
  Short Portable Mental
    Status Questionnaire,
    42-44
Cold remedies, 36
Colon, 250
Columns of Morgagni, 271
Comfort during physical
    examination, 55
Concentration, general
    survey, 92
Concha, 151
Conduction system of
    heart, 219-223
Conductive deafness, 173
Condyloid joint, 307
Confusional state, 363
Congestive heart failure
  nutrient deficiency, 72
  presentation in elderly, 8
Conjunctiva, 132, 141
Constipation, 264-265, 271
Continence, 39, 40
Convulsion, 74

Cooper's suspensory
    ligaments, 179, 180
Coordination, 340
Coping ability, 5
Cornea, 134, 142
Corneal light reflex, 139
Corona, 266
Corpora cavernosa, 266
Corpus spongiosum, 266
Corrigan pulse, 229
Cortical sensation, 343
Corticosteroids, 36
Costal angle, 195
Costal cartilage, 200
Costodiaphragmatic recess,
    199
Cover-uncover test, 139
Crackle, 207
Cranial nerves, 328
  anatomy and physiology,
    332-333
  functional assessment,
    338-339
Cranium, 118
Creatinine, 358
Creatinine clearance, 359
Crust, 100
Culture, vaginal, 291-293
Cyst, 99

D

Decompression of
    bladder, 371
Decongestants, 365
Deep tendon reflexes,
    343-345
Delayed wound healing, 74
Delirium
  common manifestation of
    illness, 7
  transient urinary
    incontinence, 363
Dementia, 44
Dentition of permanent
    teeth, 157

Depression, 74
  Beck Depression Inventory,
      49-51
  dementia *versus,* 44
  Geriatric Depression
      Scale, 52
  presentation in elderly, 9
Dermatitis, 69
Dermatomes, 335-336
Dermis, 102, 104
Descending colon, 250
Developmental norms, 6
Diabetes insipidus, 158
Diabetes mellitus, 158
Diaphragm, 195
Diaphragmatic excursion,
    204
Diarrhea, 74
Diarthrosis, 307
Diastole, 240
Diastolic blood pressure, 224
Dicyclomine hydrochloride,
    365, 367
Diencephalon, 331
Dietary analysis, 68-75
Digestive enzymes, 252
Disability, 4
Discriminatory sensation,
    343
Disease
  altered presentation and
      response to, 6-9
  nature of, 4
Disopyramide, 365
Disorientation, 73
Distal convoluted tubule, 251
Distant vision, 137
Diuretics, 364
Dorsalis pedis pulse, 227
Dowager's hump, 121
Doxazosin, 365
Doxepin, 367
Dressing habits, 38, 40
Drug intoxication, 11

Drug therapy
  effects that may affect
      assessment, 36
  oral manifestations, 158
  urinary incontinence, 364,
      366-368
Drusen, 135
Dry mouth, 178
Dry skin, 112
Dry smear, 293
Dullness, 60
Duodenum, 249

E
Ear
  anatomy and physiology,
      150-153
  assessment, 159-162
  Hearing Disability
      Inventory, 175
  hearing loss, 176
  hearing tests, 172-174
  otoscopic examination, 171
  review of systems, 29-30
Earlobe, 150-152
Eccrine glands, 109
Ectropion, 132
Edema, 70, 73, 231, 232
Egophony, 210
Ejaculatory duct, 267-269
Elbow range of motion, 319
Electrical conduction
      system, 219-223
Electrocardiogram, 223
Emotional stress
  acute confusional states, 11
  impact on immune system,
      5
  oral manifestations, 158
Endocardium, 215
Endocrine disorders
  acute confusional states, 11
  pruritus, 105
Endocrine system, 34
Entropion, 132

Environment
  acute confusional states,
    10-12
  interrelationship between
    physical and
    psychosocial aspects of
    aging, 2
  tailoring assessment to older
    person, 12-14
Enzyme laboratory
    values, 359
Epicardium, 215
Epidermal appendages,
    103-104
Epidermis, 95, 102, 103
Epithalamus, 331
Equilibrium, 340-341
Erythrocyte sedimentation
    rate, 358
Esophageal reflux, 263-264
Esophagus, 246
Estrogen supplementation
    therapy, 367
Ethmoid bone, 153
Eversion, 310
Excessive urine
    production, 363
Excoriation, 101
Extension, 310
External auditory canal, 150,
    152
External auditory meatus, 151
External ear, 150-152
External nose, 153
Extraocular muscles, 136,
    137, 139
Eye, 131-149
  accommodation, 143
  cataract, 145
  client teaching, 148
  external, 131-134
  extraocular muscles, 136,
    137, 139
  inspection, 140-143
  internal, 134-135

Eye—cont'd
  ophthalmoscopic, 146-147
  retinal vessels, 144-145
  review of systems, 29
  signs of nutrient
    deficiency, 70-71
  vision assessment, 136-137
Eyebrow, 132, 140
Eyelid, 131-132, 140

F
Face
  anatomy and physiology,
    118-120
  general survey, 90-91
  inspection, 123-125
  sialadenitis, 129
Facial nerve, 333
  assessment, 124, 169
  taste, 156
Fall prevention, 323-324
Fallopian tube, 281
Family APGAR, 52-53
Family history, 27
Family profile, 24
Fatigue, 74
Feeding habits, 39, 40
Female
  genitalia, 277-303
    anal sphincter tone, 302
    anus and rectum, 282
    atrophic vaginitis, 303
    bimanual examination,
      294-301
    external, 277-278,
      283-286
    internal, 278-281
    pelvic examination,
      286-290
    rectovaginal examination,
      302
    speculum examination,
      290
    vaginal smears and
      cultures, 291-293

Female—cont'd
  urinary incontinence,
    368-376
    overflow, 371
    stress, 368-372
    urge, 372-376
Femoral nerve, 334
Femoral pulse, 227
Fever, 158
Fibrosis, 305
Finger range of motion, 320
Finger-to-finger test, 341
Finger-to-nose test, 340
First heart sound, 218, 238
Fissure, 102
Flatness, 60
Flexion, 310
Follicular keratosis, 69
Food diary, 75
Food Guide Pyramid, 86
Foot
  assessment, 311-312
  care guidelines, 313
Foreskin, 266
Fourth heart sound, 219,
    240
Frail elderly
  mechanical loading and
    support surfaces, 391
  position during health
    history interview, 20
  urinary incontinence,
    378-382
Fremitus, 203
Frenulum, 156
Friction, pressure sore risk,
    106, 387
Friction rub, 207
Frontal bone, 153
Functional status, 37-40
  effect of selected
    variables, 3
  nature of disease and
    disability, 4

G

Gait, 339-340
Gallbladder, 250
Gardnerella, 293
Gastrointestinal tract
  anatomy and physiology,
    246-250
  review of systems, 32
General survey, 88-94
Genitalia
  female, 277-303
    anal sphincter tone, 302
    anus and rectum, 282
    atrophic vaginitis, 303
    bimanual examination,
      294-301
    external, 277-278,
      283-286
    internal, 278-281
    pelvic examination,
      286-290
    rectovaginal examination,
      302
    speculum examination,
      290
    vaginal smears and
      cultures, 291-293
  male, 266-276
    anus and rectum,
      270-271
    assessment, 272-275
    benign prostatic
      hyperplasia, 276
    penis, 266-267, 268
    prostate gland, 269-270
    scrotum, 267-269
  review of systems, 33
Geriatric Depression Scale,
    48, 52
Glands, 108
Glans penis, 266
Glaucoma, 134
Gliding joint, 307
Globe, 132
Glomerulus, 251

Glossitis, 71
Glossopharyngeal nerve, 156, 168, 169, 333
Glucagon, 250
Glucose laboratory values, 358
Gonococcal culture specimen, 292-293
Graphesthesia, 343
Gray matter, 328
Great vessels, 217
Grooming, 90
Guided reminiscence, 16
Gums, 166
Gynecomastia, 182

H
Hair, 108
    assessment, 115
    signs of nutrient deficiency, 69
Hard palate, 154-155, 168
Head
    anatomy and physiology, 118-120
    inspection, 123-125
    review of systems, 29
Head lice, 113
Health history, 19-35
    client factors, 21-23
    drugs and associated effects, 36
    format, 23-35
    sample write-up, 349-354
    symptom analysis factors, 23
Hearing Disability Inventory, 175
Hearing loss
    client teaching, 176
    effect on history taking, 21
    Hearing Disability Inventory, 175
Hearing tests, 172-174

Heart, 214-243
    anatomy and physiology, 214-218
    auscultation, 236-240
    blood pressure, 227-230
    cardiac cycle, 218-219
    conduction system, 219-223
    heart sounds, 219, 220-222
    hypertension, 241
    review of systems, 31-32
    risk factors for cardiac disease, 242
    signs of nutrient deficiency, 72
Heart disease
    client teaching, 242
    risk factors, 10
Heart murmur, 219, 220-222, 240
Heart rate, 224
Heart sounds, 217-222
Heel-to-shin test, 341
Height
    changes in vertebral column, 121
    measurement, 76
Helix, 151
Hematocrit, 358
Hematology laboratory values, 358
Hematopoietic system, 29
Hemoglobin, 225, 358
Hemorrhoids, 271
Hepatic disease, 104
Hepatic flexure, 250
Hepatojugular reflux, 235
Hepatomegaly, 72
Herpes zoster, 112
Hinge joint, 307
Hip range of motion, 320-321
Histamine receptor antagonists, 36
Homeostasis, 4-5
Hormone laboratory values, 359

Houston's valves, 271
Hygiene
    general survey, 90
    skin assessment, 109-110
Hyoid bone, 156
Hyperresonance, 60
Hypertension, 224-225, 241
Hyperthyroidism, 9
Hypnotics
    effects that may affect
        assessment, 36
    transient urinary
        incontinence, 364
Hypodermis, 104
Hypoglossal nerve, 156, 167,
    333
Hyporeflexia, 73
Hypothalamus, 331
Hypothyroidism, 9

I

Ileum, 249
Illness, lack of standard
    norms, 5-6
Imipramine, 367
Immune system, 5
Incus, 152
Index of Independence in
    Activities of Daily
    Living, 38
Infection
    acute confusional states, 10
    candidiasis, 158
    presentation in elderly, 8
    transient urinary
        incontinence, 363
Inferior vena cava, 217
Influenza prevention, 212
Information-Memory-
    Concentration
    Test, 41-44, 47
Inframammary ridge, 182
Inguinal canal, 267
Inguinal lymph node, 263
Inguinal ring, 274

Inner ear, 153
Inspection, 56-57
    abdomen, 253-254
    breast, 182-186
    ear, 159-160
    eye, 141-143
    foot, 312
    general survey, 88, 89, 90
    head and face, 123-124
    mouth and oropharynx,
        166-167
    musculoskeletal system,
        314-315
    neck, 125-126
    nose, 163
    ocular structures, 140
    skin, 109-110
Insulin, 250
Intake patterns and practices,
    75
Integument
    cross-section of skin, 102
    herpes zoster, 112
    inspection, 109-110
    pressure ulcer, 105, 108,
        117, 383-392
        bony prominences
            vulnerable to pressure,
            115
        Braden Scale, 106-107
        education programs,
            389-390
        etiology, 108
        management algorithm,
            390-391
        mechanical loading and
            support surfaces,
            388-389, 391-392
        nutrient deficiency, 70
        risk assessment tools and
            risk factors, 385, 386
        skin care and early
            treatment, 385-388,
            392
        staging, 114

Integument—cont'd
  pruritus, 104, 105
  review of systems, 28
  skin lesions
    abnormal, 112-113
    normal, 103
    primary, 96-99
    secondary, 100-102
  xerosis, 116-117
Intercostal muscles, 195
Interview, 15-53
  adapting interviewing
      techniques, 15-19, 20
  cognitive/affective status
      assessment, 41-50
    Beck Depression
      Inventory, 49-51
    Mini-Mental State
      Exam, 44-45
    Short Blessed Test, 47
    Short Portable Mental
      Status Questionnaire,
      42-44
  functional assessment,
      37-40
  health history, 19-35
    client factors, 21-23
    drugs and associated
      effects, 36
    format, 23-35
    symptom analysis
      factors, 23
  social assessment, 50-52
Inversion, 310
Iris, 134, 142
Irradiation, oral
      manifestations, 158
Islets of Langerhans, 250

J

Jejunum, 249
Joint
  classification, 307
  general survey, 91
  movement, 310

Joint—cont'd
  range of motion assessment,
      317-322
Judgment, general survey, 92
Jugular vein, 224
Jugular venous pressure,
      233-235

K

Katz Index of Activities of
      Daily Living, 37-40
Keloid, 101
Keratin, 95
Keratomalacia, 70
Kidney, 251, 261-262
Knee height measurement, 80
Knee range of motion, 321
Koilonychia, 72
Kyphosis, 200

L

Labia majora, 277, 283
Labia minora, 277
Labile pulse, 229
Laboratory values, 358-359
  normal *versus* abnormal,
      5-6
Labyrinth, 153
Lacrimal system, 133-134
Large intestine, 249-250
Lens, 134
Lethargy, 74
Lichen sclerosus et
      atrophicus, 282
Lichenification, 100
Light touch, 341
Lip, 71, 154
Liver, 250
  palpation, 259
  percussion, 256-257
Living environment
      profile, 24
Loop of Henle, 251
Lumbar plexus, 334

Lumbar spine range of
    motion, 318
Lung, 194-213
    anatomic and thoracic
        landmarks, 195-196,
        197
    assessment, 200-210
    breath sounds, 206-207,
        209
    influenza prevention, 212
    pneumonia, 211
    respiration, 198-200
Lymph nodes
    breast, 181-182, 188
    head and neck, 122-123
    inguinal, 263

M

Macula, 135, 145
Macule, 96
Male
    genitalia, 266-276
        anus and rectum, 270-271
        assessment, 272-275
        benign prostatic
            hyperplasia, 276
        penis, 266-267, 268
        prostate gland, 269-270
        scrotum, 267-269
    urinary incontinence,
        376-378
Malignant melanoma, 112
Malleus, 152
Malnutrition, 158
Mammary glands, 179-181
Mandible, 119
Manubriosternal junction, 195
Mass in breast, 188, 192
Maxilla, 119
Mechanical loading and
        support surfaces,
        388-389, 391-392
Mediastinum, 196
Medulla oblongata, 330
Melanin, 103

Melanocyte, 95, 103
Membranous labyrinth, 153
Memory, mental status
        assessment, 93
Mental disorders, 73
Mental status, 34-35, 88-94
Metabolic disturbances, 10-11
Methyldopa, 36
Midarm circumference, 80
Midarm muscle area, 83
Midbrain, 330
Midclavicular lines, 196
Middle ear, 152
Midposition uterus, 298
Midspinal line, 196
Midsternal line, 196
Mid-upper arm
        circumference, 81
Mini-Mental State Exam, 41,
        44-46
Minimum Data Set, 35
Mitral valve, 215-216
Mixed incontinence, 362
MMSE; see Mini-Mental State
        Exam
Mobility deficit
    pressure ulcer risk, 106,
        391
    transient urinary
        incontinence, 364
Modesty during physical
        examination, 55
Moisture, pressure sore
        risk, 106
Mons pubis, 277, 283
Mood, 93
Mouth
    anatomy and physiology,
        154-159
    assessment, 166-169
    oral health care, 177-178
    review of systems, 30
    sialadenitis, 129
    signs of nutrient deficiency,
        71

Murmur, 220-222
Muscle strength screening,
    315-317
Muscle wasting, 72, 73, 314
Muscles, 308-309
    abdominal, 251
    extraocular, 136, 137, 139
    female perineum, 279-280
    intercostal, 195
    papillary, 216-217
    thoracic, 195
Musculoskeletal system,
    304-325
    anatomy and physiology,
        305-311
        bones, 306
        joints, 307, 310
        muscles, 308-309
    ballottement, 324
    bulge sign, 324-325
    fall prevention, 323-324
    foot assessment, 311-312
    foot care guidelines, 313
    functional status after
        injury, 3
    inspection, 314-315
    muscle strength screening,
        315-317
    osteoporosis, 325
    range of motion assessment,
        317-322
    review of systems, 33-34
    signs of nutrient deficiency,
        73
Myocardial infarction, 8
Myocardium, 215

N

Nails, 108
    assessment, 115
    signs of nutrient
        deficiency, 72
Narcotics, 36

Nasal cavity
    anatomy and physiology,
        153-154, 155
    assessment, 163-165
Nasal fossa, 153
Nasal septum, 153
Nasolabial folds, 119
Nasolacrimal duct, 153
Nausea, 74
Near vision, 138
Neck
    anatomy and physiology,
        120-123
    inspection and palpation,
        125-129
    review of systems, 31
Nephritis, 158
Nephron, 251
Neurologic system, 326-348
    Alzheimer's disease, 348
    anatomy and physiology,
        327-338
        brain, 327-329
        brainstem, 330-331
        cranial nerves, 332-333
        sensory dermatomes,
            335-336
        spinal cord, 328,
            337-338
    assessment, 338-347
        balance, 339-341
        cranial nerves, 338-339
        percussion hammer,
            344-345
        reflexes, 343, 345-347
        sensory examination,
            341-343
    review of systems, 34
    signs of nutrient deficiency,
        73-74
Nipple, 180, 181, 184
Nitrate, 36
Nitrite, 36
Nodule, 97

Nonsteroidal antiinflammatory drugs, 36
Norton Scale, 385, 386
Nose
  anatomy and physiology, 153-154, 155
  assessment, 163-165
  review of systems, 30
Nursing assessment, 1-14
  acute confusional states, 10-12
  altered presentation of diseases, 6-9
  decreased efficiency of homeostasis, 4-5
  interrelationship between physical and psychosocial aspects of aging, 2-4
  lack of standards for health and illness norms, 5-6
  nature of disease and disability, 4
  nursing foundations, 1-2
  tailoring assessment to older person, 12-14
Nutrition screening, 64-75
  anthropometric measurement, 67-68
  biochemical measurement, 68
  clinical examination, 69, 70-74
  dietary analysis, 68-75
  Nutrition Screening Initiative Checklist, 66-67
  risk factors associated with poor nutritional status, 65
Nutrition Screening Initiative Checklist, 66-67

Nutritional assessment, 62-87
  anthropometric measurement, 75-87
    height, 76-77
    knee height, 80
    midarm circumference, 80
    mid-upper arm circumference, 81
    triceps skinfold thickness, 82-85
    weight, 78-79
  Food Guide Pyramid, 86
  nutrition screening, 64-75
    anthropometric measurement, 67-68
    biochemical measurement, 68
    clinical examination, 69, 70-74
    dietary analysis, 68-75
    Nutrition Screening Initiative Checklist, 66-67
    risk factors associated with poor nutritional status, 65
Nutritional deficiency
  acute confusional states, 11
  pressure sore risk, 106

O

Observation, general survey, 89
Occupational profile, 24
Ocular orbit, 131
Oculomotor nerve, 137, 332
Odontomyces viscosus, 158
Odor, 56-57
Oil glands, 104
Olfactory bulb, 153
Olfactory function, 164
Olfactory nerve, 153, 332
Ophthalmoplegia, 73

Ophthalmoscopic examination, 146-147
Opiates, 365
Optic disc, 135, 144
Optic nerve, 135, 332
Oral cavity
  anatomy and physiology, 154-159
  assessment, 166-169
  oral health care, 177-178
  review of systems, 30
  sialadenitis, 129
  signs of nutrient deficiency, 71
Oral health care, 177-178
Oral mucosa
  assessment, 165
  increase in tissue friability, 158
Orbit, 131
Orbital fat, 131
Organ of Corti, 153
Orientation, general survey, 91-92
Oropharynx
  anatomy and physiology, 154-159
  assessment, 166-169
Osteoporosis, 305
  documentation, 325
  oral manifestations, 158
Otoscope, 164
Otoscopic examination, 171
Ovary, 281, 296
Overflow incontinence, 362
  female, 371
  male, 376-378
  surgical management, 368
Over-the-counter agents, 365
Oviduct, 281
Oxybutynin chloride, 367
Oxygen partial pressure, 359

P

P wave, 223
Pain
  assessment, 342
  effect on history taking, 22
  during palpation, 58
Palatine arch, 155
Palatine tonsil, 155
Pallor, 70, 74
Palpation, 58-59
  abdomen, 258-263
  Bartholin's glands, 285
  breast, 186-191
  carotid artery, 226
  foot, 312
  lacrimal gland, 140
  sinuses, 165
  Skene's duct, 284
  temporal artery, 124
  thoracic, 202
  thyroid, 126-129
  tongue and floor of mouth, 169
  uterus, 294-301
Palpebral fissure, 119, 132
Pancreas, 250-251
Pap smear, 291-292
Papillary muscles, 216-217
Papule, 96
Paradoxical pulse, 229
Parietal pericardium, 199
Parietal pleura, 199
Parotid gland, 155, 156
Pars flaccida, 152
Pars tensa, 152
Past health status, 27
Patch, 96
Patellar reflex, 347
Pathologic reflexes, 347
Pediculosis capitis, 113
Pediculosis corporis, 113
Pelvic examination, 286-290
Pelvic prolapse, 374-375
Penis, 266-267, 268, 272

Perceptive deafness, 174
Percussion, 59, 60
  abdomen, 255-258
  chest, 203, 208-209
Percussion hammer, 344-345
Perianal area, 274
Pericardial friction rub, 241
Pericardium, 215
Perifollicular hemorrhage, 70
Perineum, 279, 284, 285
Periodontal disease, 177
Periodontal structures, 156
Peripheral chemoreceptor, 199
Peripheral circulation,
    223-226
Peripheral nervous system,
    327
Peripheral neuropathy, 74
Peripheral pulses, 224
Pernicious anemia, 158
Petechiae, 69
Phenylpropanoline, 367
Photophobia, 71
Physical assessment, 54-61
  auscultation, 59-61
  comfort and modesty
      during, 55
  equipment, 56, 57
  examination approach and
      sequence, 54-55
  general guidelines, 55-56
  inspection, 56-57
  palpation, 58-59
  percussion, 59, 60
  sample write-up, 354-357
  urinary incontinence, 361
Physical frailty, 4
Pinguecula, 132
Pinna, 150
Pitting edema, 232
Pituitary gland, 331
Pivot joint, 307
Plantar reflex, 347
Plaque, 97

Pleural friction rub, 207
Pneumonia, 8, 211
Point localization, 343
Polyp, rectal, 271
Polypharmacy, 6
Pons, 330
Popliteal pulse, 227
Position awareness, 342
Positioning device, 388
Posterior chamber, 134
Posterior tibial pulse, 227
Potassium
  effects that may affect
      assessment, 36
  laboratory values, 358
Potassium hydroxide
      procedure, 293
P-R interval, 223
Prazosin, 365
Prepuce, 266
Presbycusis, 153, 176
Present health status, 25-26
Pressure ulcer, 105, 108, 117,
    383-392
  bony prominences
      vulnerable to pressure,
      115
  Braden Scale, 106-107
  education programs,
      389-390
  etiology, 108
  management algorithm,
      390-391
  mechanical loading and
      support surfaces,
      388-389, 391-392
  nutrient deficiency, 70
  risk assessment tools and
      risk factors, 385, 386
  skin care and early
      treatment, 385-388,
      392
  staging, 114

Pressure-reducing device, 388, 389
Prolapse, pelvic, 374-375
Pronation, 310
Propantheline bromide, 367
Proprioception, 340
Prostate gland
    anatomy and physiology, 269-270
    assessment, 275
    benign prostatic hyperplasia, 276
Proximal convoluted tubule, 251
Pruritus, 104
Pudendal nerve, 334
Pudendum, 277
Pulmonary abnormalities, 10
Pulmonary artery, 217
Pulmonary vein, 218
Pulmonic valve, 216
Pulsus alternans, 228
Pulsus bigeminus, 228
Pulsus bisferiens, 228
Pulsus differens, 229
Pulsus paradoxus, 229
Pulsus trigeminus, 229
Pupil, 143
Purpura, 70
Pustule, 99

Q
QRS complex, 223

R
Radial pulse, 227
Range of motion assessment, 317-322
Rapid alternating movements, 340
Recreation/leisure profile, 24
Rectal ampulla, 270-271
Rectal polyp, 271
Rectovaginal examination, 302

Rectum, 270-271
    assessment, 275
    female, 282
Rectus abdominis, 251
Red reflex, 143
Reduced energy level, 22
Reflex arc, 337, 338
Reflexes, 343-347
Reminiscence, 22
Renal disease, 104
Reserpine, 36
Resident Assessment Instrument, 35
Resident Assessment Protocols, 35
Resonance, 60
Respiration, 198-200
Respiratory rate, 201
Respiratory system, 194-213
    anatomic and thoracic landmarks, 195-196, 197
    assessment, 200-210
    breath sounds, 206-207, 209
    influenza prevention, 212
    pneumonia, 211
    respiration, 198-200
    review of systems, 31
Retina, 134-135, 145
Retinal vessels, 135, 144
Retroflexed uterus, 301
Retroverted uterus, 299
Review of systems, 27-35
Ribs, 194, 200
Rinne test, 162
Rotation, 310

S
Sacral plexus, 334
Saddle joint, 307
Salicylates, 36
Saliva, 118-119, 156
Salivary gland, 118-119, 129, 156

Scabies, 113
Scale, 100
Scalp, 123
Scaphoid fossa, 151
Scapular lines, 196
Scar, 101
Sciatic nerve, 334
Sclera, 134, 141
Sclerosis of valve
      leaflets, 224
Scratch test, 254
Screening
   muscle strength, 315-317
   nutrition, 64-75
      anthropometric
         measurement, 67-68
      biochemical
         measurement, 68
      clinical examination, 69,
         70-74
      dietary analysis, 68-75
      Nutrition Screening
         Initiative Checklist,
         66-67
      risk factors associated
         with poor nutritional
         status, 65
Scrotum, 267-269, 272-273
Sebaceous gland, 108
Sebaceous hyperplasia, 103
Seborrheic dermatitis, 70, 112
Seborrheic keratosis, 103
Second heart sound, 218-219,
      238-239
Sedative hypnotics
   effects that may affect
      assessment, 36
   transient urinary
      incontinence, 364
Sedimentation rate, 358
Self breast exam, 192-193
Semicircular canal, 153
Semilunar valve, 215, 216
Seminal vesicle, 267-269
Senile ectasia, 103

Senile keratosis, 112
Senile lentigines, 103
Sensorineural loss, 174
Sensory dermatomes, 335-336
Sensory examination, 341-343
Shear, pressure sore risk, 105,
      387
Short Blessed Scale, 41-44,
      47
Short Portable Mental Status
      Questionnaire, 41,
      42-44
Shoulder range of motion,
      319
Sialadenitis, 129
Simple reflex arc, 337, 338
Simple stress urinary
      incontinence, 368-370
Sinuses, 155
   palpation, 165
   review of systems, 30
Sinusitis, 170
Skeletal muscle, 305
Skeleton, 306
Skene's glands, 278, 284
Skin
   cross-section, 102
   herpes zoster, 112
   inspection, 109-110
   lesions
      abnormal, 112-113
      normal, 103
      primary, 96-99
      secondary, 100-102
   pressure ulcer, 105, 108,
      117, 383-392
      bony prominences
         vulnerable to pressure,
         111
      Braden Scale, 106-107
      education programs,
         389-390
      etiology, 104
      management algorithm,
         390-391

Skin—cont'd
  pressure ulcer—cont'd
    mechanical loading and
      support surfaces,
      388-389, 391-392
    nutrient deficiency, 70
    risk assessment tools and
      risk factors, 385, 386
    skin care and early
      treatment, 385-388,
      392
    staging, 114
  pruritus, 105, 108
  signs of nutrient deficiency,
    69-70
  thoracic, 201
  xerosis, 116-117
Skin lesions
  abnormal, 112-113
  normal, 103
  primary, 96-99
  secondary, 100-102
Skin tags, 103
Skull, 119
Sleep disturbances, 74
Small intestine, 249
Smear, vaginal, 291-293
Social assessment, 48, 51
Soft palate, 155, 168
Specific gravity, 359
Speculum examination,
    287-290
Speech, general survey, 91
Spermatic cord, 267
Sphenoid bone, 153
Spinal accessory nerve, 125,
    333
Spinal cord, 328, 337-338
Spinal nerves, 328, 338
Spleen, 251
  palpation, 260
  percussion, 257-258
Splenic flexure, 250
Squamous cell carcinoma, 112
S-T segment, 223

Stapes, 152
Stature percentiles, 77
Stensen's duct, 155, 156
Stereognosis, 343
Sternocleidomastoid
    muscle, 120
Sternum, 194
Stomach, 246-249
Stomatitis, 71
Stool impaction, 364
Straight leg-raising test, 322
Stress
  acute confusional states, 11
  impact on immune system,
    5
  oral manifestations, 158
Stress incontinence, 362
  female, 368-372
  surgical management, 368
Stretch receptor, 200
Subcutaneous fatty tissue,
    102
Subcutaneous layer, 108
Sublingual gland, 155, 156
Submandibular gland, 155,
    156
Submaxillary gland, 156
Summation gallop, 219
Superficial skin reflexes, 262
Superficial temporal pulse,
    227
Superior vena cava, 217
Supination, 310
Suprasternal notch, 195
Suture, 307
Sympatholytics, 365
Sympathomimetics, 365
Symphysis, 307
Symptom analysis factors, 23
Synarthrosis, 307
Synchondrosis, 307
Syndesmosis, 307
Systole, 240
Systolic blood pressure, 224

T

T wave, 223
Tachycardia, 72, 229
Tactile fremitus, 203
Tail of Spence, 179, 180
Taste bud, 156
Telangiectasia, 99
Temporal artery, 120, 124
Temporomandibular joint, 318
Terazosin, 365
Testis, 267, 272-273
Testosterone, 269
Thalamus, 331
Third heart sound, 219, 239
Thoracic aorta, 251
Thoracic expansion, 202
Thoracic muscles, 195
Thorax, 194-213
    anatomic landmarks,
        195-196, 197
    assessment, 200-210
    client teaching, 212
    pneumonia, 211
    respiration, 198-200
Though content and
        processes, 93
Throat
    anatomy and physiology,
        154-159
    assessment, 166-169
    review of systems, 30
Thrombosis, 230
Thumb range of motion, 320
Thyroid, 121-122, 126-129
Thyroid-stimulating
        hormone, 359
Thyroxine, 122
Toe range of motion, 321
Toileting, 39, 40
Tongue, 155-156
    assessment, 167
    signs of nutrient
        deficiency, 71
Tonsil, 168

Tooth, 156
    assessment, 167
    dentition, 157
Tooth enamel, 156
Touch, 17
Trachea, 121, 126, 198, 202
Tracheobronchial tree, 198
Tragus, 151
Transfer, 39, 40
Transverse colon, 250
Trapezius muscle, 120
Triangular fossa, 151
Triceps reflex, 346
Triceps skinfold thickness,
        82-85
Trichomonas vaginalis, 293
Tricuspid valve, 215
Tricyclic antidepressants
    effects that may affect
        assessment, 36
    urinary incontinence, 367
Trigeminal nerve, 124, 332
Trigeminal pulse, 229
Trihexyphenidyl, 365
Triiodothyronine, 122
Trochlear nerve, 137, 332
TSH; *see* Thyroid-stimulating
        hormone
Tumor, 98
Tuning fork, 161-162,
        172-174
Turgor, 69
24-hour recall, 68-75
Two-point discrimination, 343
Tympanic membrane, 152,
        160
Tympany, 60

U

Ulcer, pressure, 105, 108,
        383-392
    bony prominences
        vulnerable to
        pressure, 111
    Braden Scale, 106-107

Ulcer, pressure—cont'd
  education programs,
    389-390
  etiology, 105
  management algorithm,
    390-391
  mechanical loading and
    support surfaces,
    388-389, 391-392
  nutrient deficiency, 70
  risk assessment tools and
    risk factors, 385, 386
  skin care and early
    treatment, 385-388,
    392
  staging, 114
Upper respiratory system,
    150-178
  ear
    anatomy and physiology,
      150-153
    assessment, 159-162
    Hearing Disability
      Inventory, 175
    hearing loss, 176
    hearing tests, 172-174
    otoscopic examination,
      171
  mouth and oropharynx
    anatomy and physiology,
      154-159
    assessment, 166-169
    oral health care, 177-178
  nose and nasal cavity
    anatomy and physiology,
      153-154, 155
    assessment, 163-165
Ureter, 251
Urethra, 251
Urethral meatus
  female, 278, 283-284
  male, 266, 272
Urge incontinence, 362
  female, 372-376
  surgical management, 368

Uric acid, 359
Urinalysis, 361-362
Urinary incontinence, 360-382
  client management,
    360-368
  female, 368-376
  male, 376-378
  nursing home client,
    378-382
Urinary system, 32
Urinary tract infection
  presentation in elderly, 8
  transient urinary
    incontinence, 363
Urine chemistry, 359
Uterus
  anatomy, 281
  bimanual palpation,
    294-301
Uvula, 155

V
Vagina
  anatomy, 278
  speculum examination,
    287-290
Vaginal introitus, 278, 284
Vaginal smear, 291-293
Vagus nerve, 168, 333
Varicose veins, 231
Vas deferens, 267
Vascular system, 214-243
  arterial insufficiency, 230,
    231
  blood pressure, 227-230
  carotid artery palpation,
    226
  edema, 231, 232
  hepatojugular reflux, 235
  hypertension, 241
  jugular venous pressure,
    233-235
  palpable pulses, 227
  peripheral circulation,
    223-226

Vascular system—cont'd
  thrombosis, 230
  varicose veins, 231
Venous insufficiency, 231
Venous system, 223-226
Ventral ramus, 334
Ventricle, 214
Vertebra prominens, 195
Vesicle, 98
Vesicular sounds, 209
Vestibule, 153, 278
Vibration, 342
Visceral pericardium, 199
Vision assessment, 136-137
Vision loss, 3
Visual acuity, 137
Visual disturbance, 21
Visual fields, 138
Vitamin deficiencies, 158
Voice test, 161
Vulva, 277

W

Watch-tick test, 161
Water-hammer pulse, 229
Weakness, 73
Weber test, 161

Weight, 78, 79
Wet prep, 293
Wharton's duct, 155, 156
Wheal, 97
Wheelchair-bound patient
  mechanical loading and
      support surfaces,
      391-392
  position during health
      history interview, 18
Wheeze, 206
Whispered pectoriloquy, 210
White matter, 328
Wrist range of motion, 320

X

Xerosis, 69, 116-117
Xerostomia, 159

Y

Yesavage Geriatric Depression
      Scale, 48, 52

Z

Zona hemorrhoidalis, 271
Zygomatic bone, 119